LOST
ENCYCLOPEDIA OF
NATURAL
REMEDIES

OVER 1000 HOMEMADE ANTIBIOTICS, HERBS AND REMEDIES FOR HEALING WITHOUT PILLS

Batbara O'Neil & Hulda Regehr Clark

By

Andrew Clapham &

Melody Gerald, Ph.D

GREENRAVE
PUBLICATION

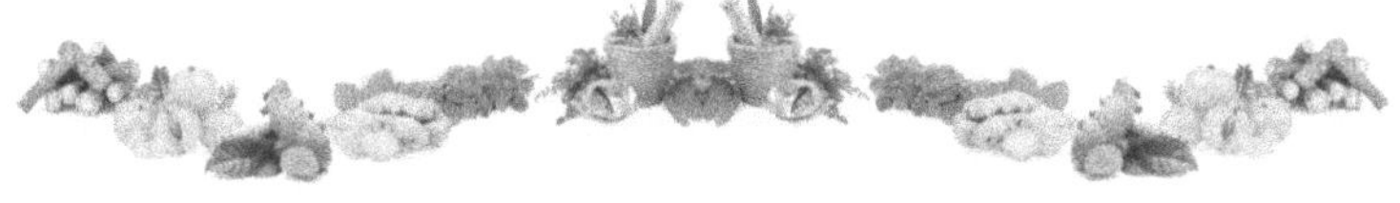

CONTENT

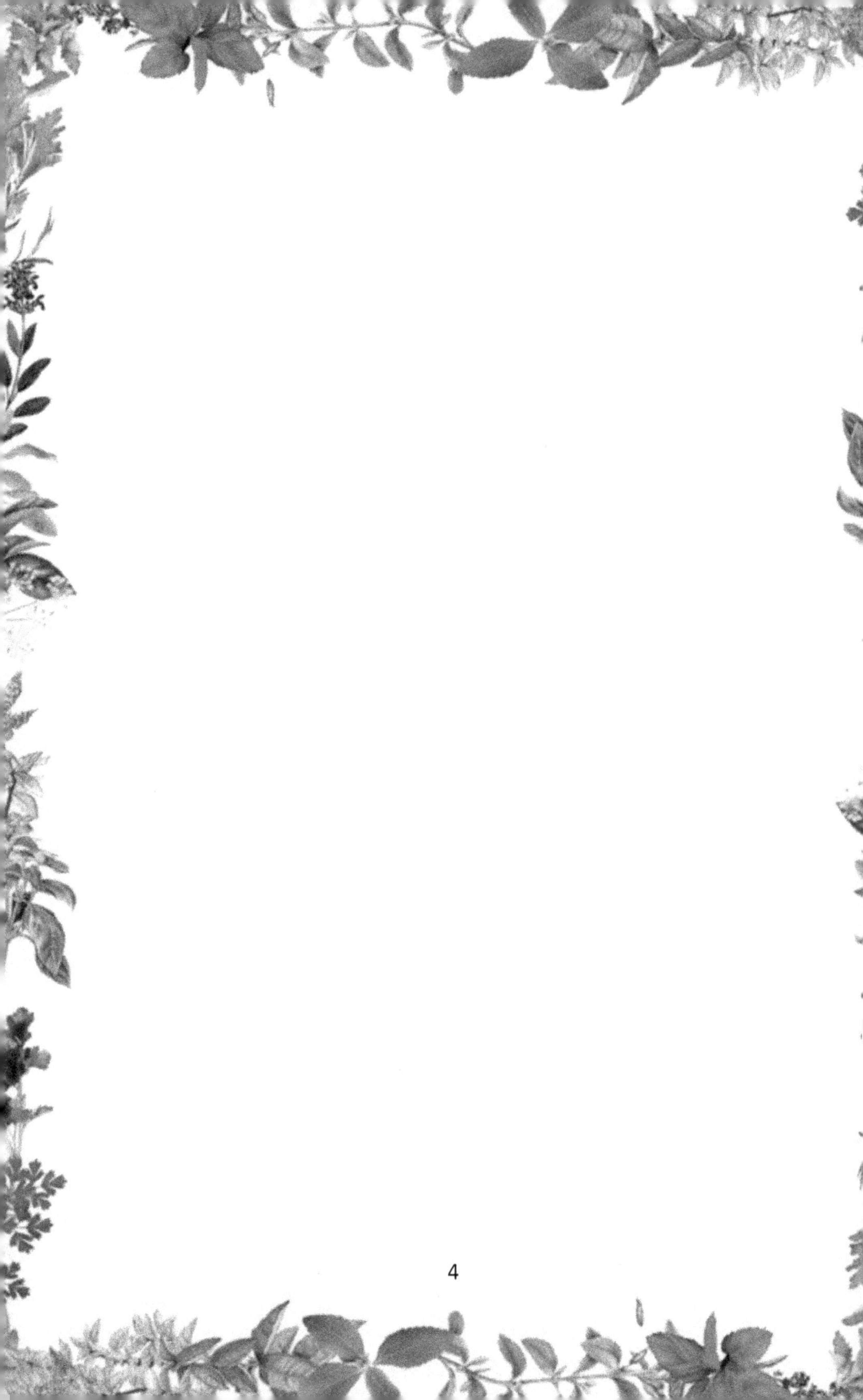

INTRODUCTION

Welcome to "Unveiling Nature's Arsenal," a stellar companion workbook purposefully designed to enhance your journey through the wisdom of "The Lost Book of Natural Remedies" by Amanda Adams. In her groundbreaking book, Adams explores the incredible efficacy of natural remedies for combating various ailments and fostering self-healing.

This workbook is crafted with the intention of guiding you through reflective exercises and practical activities. "Unveiling Nature's Arsenal" serves as your personal companion on the path to unlocking the full potential of nature's healing treasures.

Within these pages, you will discover not only a wealth of knowledge but also hands-on tools to deepen your understanding and application of the natural remedies presented in Adams' original masterpiece. Through thoughtful reflections and actionable exercises, this workbook aims to empower you to incorporate the teachings of "The Lost Book of Natural Remedies" into your daily life, fostering a holistic approach to well-being.

Prepare to embark on a transformative journey as we navigate through the bountiful offerings of nature's pharmacy, unraveling the secrets that empower us to take charge of our health and embrace the art of self-healing.

Let the exploration begin!

PART 1: FOUNDATIONS OF SELF-HEALING

At the core of our existence lies an incredible connection to nature which was designed to helps us grow, thrive and bask in the joy of our wellbeing. It is a blessing to us in such a way that helps us to improve the quality of our lives. This is to say that, without nature, we are better off at the mercy of the toxins that filter into our body systems through what we eat and drink.

Thankfully, the existence of vital roots, herbs and other natural elements help the body to fight antigens and lethal toxins that pose a threat to our entire wellness. Essentially, these gifts of nature provide us with the opportunity for self-healing. This relates to our physical, emotional and mental wellbeing.

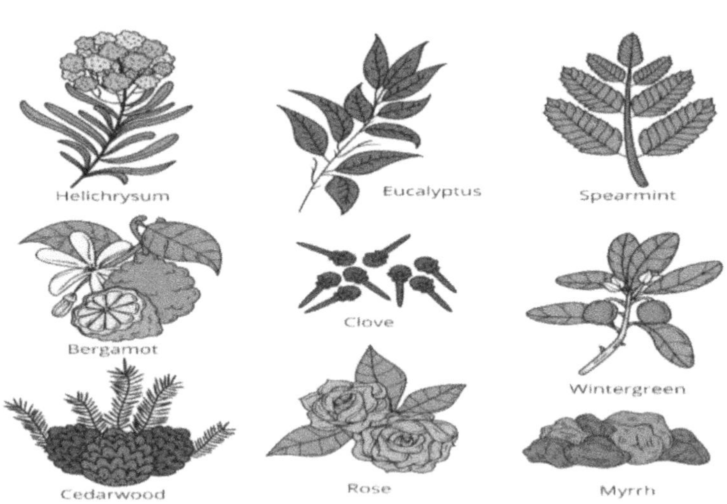

Self-healing refers to the ability of the human body of heal, repair or recover from any form of injury or imbalances that may be physical, mental and emotional. This process is orchestrated by the body's own mechanisms and natural resources, without external intervention or assistance. Self-healing is a fundamental aspect of the body's resilience and adaptive capacity to maintain or restore a state of equilibrium and well-being.

In the human body, self-healing takes various forms. Let us briefly look at them specifically:

- ❖ **Physical Self-Healing:**
  The body has mechanisms to repair damaged tissues, heal wounds, and recover from injuries. This involves processes such as inflammation, tissue regeneration, and the immune response.
- ❖ **Mental and Emotional Self-Healing:**

The mind has the capacity to adapt and recover from stress, trauma, and emotional challenges. Emotional resilience, coping mechanisms, and psychological processes contribute to mental well-being and the restoration of emotional balance.

- ❖ **Homeostasis:**
  The body continually strives to maintain internal stability and balance, a state known as homeostasis. Various physiological systems work together to regulate factors such as temperature, blood pressure, and hormone levels, contributing to overall health.

- ❖ **Immune System Function:**

The immune system plays a crucial role in self-healing by defending the body against pathogens and supporting recovery from infections. Immunological memory allows the body to mount a faster and more effective response upon subsequent exposure to familiar threats.

❖ **Adaptation:**
The body can adapt to changing environmental conditions and stressors, adjusting its functions and responses to promote survival and well-being.

Apart from being self-healing is a natural and intrinsic process, it can be influenced by lifestyle factors, environmental conditions, and individual habits. Practices that support self-healing include a nutritious diet, regular exercise, adequate sleep, stress management, and maintaining a positive mental outlook. Additionally, holistic approaches such as traditional medicine, meditation, and mindfulness can complement the body's natural ability to heal.

Understanding and nurturing the body's self-healing capacity empowers individuals to take an active role in their health and well-being, fostering a comprehensive approach to maintaining balance and vitality.

Let us look at the several ways in which nature supports and fosters the self-healing process:

Nature, in its diverse and intricate design, offers a multitude of elements that contribute to our physical, mental, and emotional well-being, providing us with ample opportunities for self-healing. Here are several ways in which nature supports and fosters the healing process:

- ❖ **Nutrient-Rich Foods:** The fruits, vegetables, herbs, and other plants found in nature provide a rich array of nutrients essential for our health. These foods offer vitamins, minerals, antioxidants, and phytochemicals that support various bodily functions, boost the immune system, and aid in the prevention and management of diseases.

- ❖ **Medicinal Herbs and Plants:** Throughout history, various cultures have relied on the healing properties of medicinal herbs and plants. Nature provides a pharmacy of botanical remedies, many of which possess anti-inflammatory, antimicrobial, and other therapeutic properties. These natural substances can be used to address a wide range of health issues, from minor ailments to chronic conditions.

- ❖ **Fresh Air and Oxygen:**
  Spending time outdoors exposes us to fresh air, rich in oxygen, which is vital for cellular function and overall well-being. Deep breathing in natural settings can enhance lung function, reduce stress, and promote a sense of calm and relaxation.

- ❖ **Sunlight and Vitamin-D**:
  Exposure to sunlight triggers the production of vitamin D in our skin, a crucial nutrient for bone health, immune function, and mental well-being. Sunlight also plays a role in regulating circadian rhythms, contributing to better sleep and overall mood.

- ❖ **Physical Activity:**
  Nature provides a natural playground for physical activity. Whether it's hiking through forests, walking along the beach, or practicing yoga in a park, engaging in physical activities outdoors promotes cardiovascular health, flexibility, and mental clarity.

- ❖ **Restorative Environments:** Nature has a unique ability to promote relaxation and stress reduction. Natural settings, such as forests, parks, or bodies of water, have been shown to lower cortisol levels, reduce anxiety, and improve mood. Access to green spaces provides an opportunity for mental rejuvenation and self-reflection.

- ❖ **Mind-Body Connection:**
  The natural environment has a profound impact on our mental state. Connecting with nature allows us to step away from the hustle and bustle of daily life, fostering mindfulness and a deeper connection with ourselves. This mind-body connection is integral to the self-healing process.
- ❖ **Biorhythms and Natural Cycles:**

Our bodies are attuned to natural rhythms and cycles, such as the circadian rhythm. Aligning our daily routines with these natural patterns supports better sleep, hormonal balance, and overall physiological harmony, contributing to self-healing.

By recognizing and embracing the gifts that nature offers, individuals can integrate these elements into their lifestyles, creating a foundation for self-healing and holistic well-being. Nature not only provides remedies for specific ailments but also nurtures a comprehensive approach to health that encompasses the physical, mental, and spiritual dimensions of our existence.

Reflections on self-healing:

- ❖ What are some instances in your life where you have noticed your body's natural ability to heal physically?

____
____
____
____
____
____

❖ How do you currently support your body's physical self-healing processes through lifestyle choices such as diet, exercise, and sleep?

____
____
____
____
____
____
____

❖ Think about a challenging emotional experience. How did you cope with and eventually overcome it?

____
____
____
____
____
____
____

❖ What activities or practices contribute to your emotional well-being and resilience?

____
____
____
____
____
____
____

❖ What are the primary sources of stress in your life, and how do they impact your overall well-being?

____
____
____
____
____
____
____
____
____
____
____
____

❖ Identify one positive habit you would like to adopt to enhance your self-healing journey. How do you plan to incorporate this habit into your daily or weekly routine?

____
____
____
____
____
____
____
____
____
____
____
____

PART II: CORE PRINCIPLES OF SELF-HEALING

The core principles of self-healing basically encompass a fundamental and integrated approach to our wellbeing which also acknowledges the interconnection between the body, soul and spirit. They are not just imperative; but, interestingly open us up to rich possibilities that abound, when we play an active role in taking care of our health.

They include:

❖ Holistic approach:

This approach acknowledges true healing. Unlike pharmaceutical products, which essentially treat signs and symptoms of certain diseases, herbs are designed to enrich the individual with full healing 3body, mind and spirit.

❖ The Power of Nature

It is believed that nature has the innate ability to give us full healing. Centuries ago, our ancestors relied on them to grow, heal and live accomplished lives.

❖ Prevention over Cure

Natural herbs basically serve to maintain good health and to prevent diseases. They can come in edible forms which could be taken routinely. Individuals are encouraged to take advantage of it for an improved wellbeing and long-term living.

❖ Personal Empowerment

The existence of these herbs radically empowers individuals to play an active role in their physical, emotional and mental

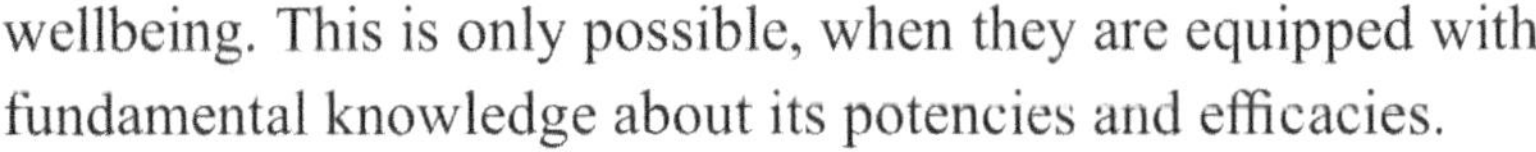

wellbeing. This is only possible, when they are equipped with fundamental knowledge about its potencies and efficacies.

Harmony with the Environment

This acknowledges the fact that humans and nature are solidly interconnected, hence, efforts should be made to leverage on this as opposed to violating it.

Benefits of Herbal Healing:

- ❖ Herbs have rich natural composition, which in fact poses less threat to human lives and has fewer side effects.
- ❖ They are easily affordable and accessible. Anyone can grow his or herbs at home.
- ❖ Herbs are incredibly versatile, and serve varieties of purposes.
- ❖ Herbs do not just treat or ameliorate the presenting ailment; but, strongly promotes the overall wellbeing of the human body through immunity, flexibility and vitality.

Reflections on Herbal Healing

- ❖ Can you recall a time when you successfully used an herbal remedy to address a specific health concern? What was the outcome?

____

____

____

____

____

____

____

____

____

____

____

____

____

❖   How did the experience influence your perspective on
    herbal healing?

____

____

____

____

____

____

____

____

____

____

____

____

❖   List three herbs commonly used in herbal healing. What
    specific health benefits are associated with each of these
    herbs?

____

____

____

____

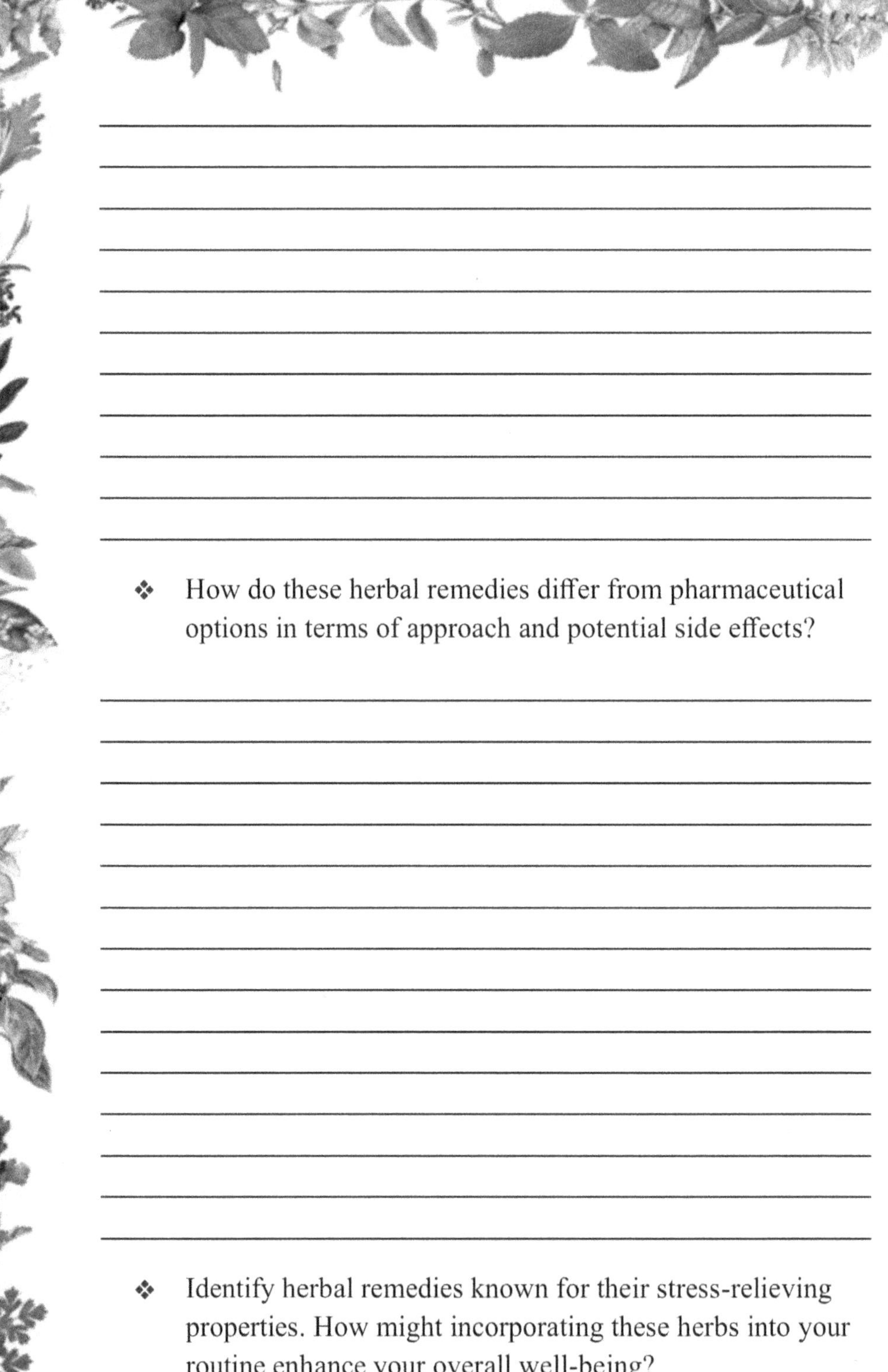

❖ How do these herbal remedies differ from pharmaceutical options in terms of approach and potential side effects?

❖ Identify herbal remedies known for their stress-relieving properties. How might incorporating these herbs into your routine enhance your overall well-being?

❖ Have you experienced the calming effects of herbal teas or supplements? Share your thoughts

❖ Research and list herbs known for boosting the immune system. How can these herbs be incorporated into your daily life to support immune health?

____

____

____

____

____

____

____

____

____

____

____

____

____

❖ In what ways do herbal remedies for immune support differ from conventional medications?

____

____

____

❖ Name two or three herbs that are traditionally used to promote digestive health. How might these herbs alleviate common digestive issues?

❖ Consider the preventive aspects of herbal remedies. In what ways can herbs support long-term health and disease prevention?

____

____

____

____

____

____

____

____

____

____

____

____

____

❖ Reflect on the long-term benefits of incorporating herbal healing into your lifestyle. How might this approach contribute to your overall well-being over time?

____

____

____

____

____

PART III: HOLISTIC APPROACHES TO COMMON DISEASES

Cardiovascular Diseases

Hypertension (High Blood Pressure)

This chapter basically explored the prevalence of hypertension (high blood pressure), and how it gradually increases as we age. Various factors that contribute to this were also delved into such as: poor dietary choices, lifestyle factors, hereditary influences etc. It is also important to note that taking cognizance of the possible symptoms, risks and root causes play vital roles in its effective management.

The chapter introduced herbal remedies as effective tools for managing hypertension. Specific herbs like golden seal, red clover, wild cherry bark, and vervain were highlighted for their potential benefits in supporting cardiovascular health. Herbal potions, such as the Golden Seal Potion and Red Clover Tea, were provided as natural remedies to incorporate into daily routines.

Additionally, lifestyle modifications were discussed as essential components of hypertension management. Suggestions included maintaining a diet free from certain elements, outdoor exercise, deep breathing, adequate rest, warm baths, and herbal teas promoting sleep. Preventative measures like regular exercise, managing salt intake, and maintaining a healthy weight were emphasized.

For individuals with persistently high blood pressure, seeking medical advice was recommended, underscoring the importance of combining herbal remedies with professional guidance for holistic hypertension management.

Reflections and Exercises:

- ❖ Reflect on your current lifestyle and identify potential factors that could contribute to high blood pressure. How might poor dietary choices, stress, and lack of rest be influencing your cardiovascular health?

____

____

____

____

____

____

____

____

____

____

____

____

____

- ❖ Have you experienced any symptoms associated with hypertension, such as morning headaches, difficulty

breathing, or dizziness? How do these symptoms impact
your daily life?

____

____

____

____

____

____

____

____

____

____

____

____

____

____

____

❖ Explore your family history for any instances of
hypertension. How might hereditary factors contribute to
your risk, and how can this awareness guide your
preventive measures?

____

____

❖ Research and list herbal remedies for hypertension
mentioned in the chapter, such as golden seal and red
clover. Which of these herbs resonates with you, and how
might you incorporate them into your routine?

❖ Experiment with creating a Golden Seal Potion or substituting your regular water intake with Red Clover Tea. How does incorporating these herbal potions into your daily routine impact your overall well-being?

❖ Evaluate your current diet and identify potential modifications to reduce salt intake, eliminate stimulants like caffeine, and incorporate heart-healthy foods. How can these dietary changes contribute to managing hypertension?

❖ Consider the importance of outdoor exercise, deep breathing, and adequate rest in hypertension management. How can you integrate these lifestyle changes into your daily routine to support cardiovascular health?

❖ Reflect on the preventative measures discussed, such as regular exercise, managing salt intake, and maintaining a healthy weight. What steps can you take to implement these measures in your life to prevent hypertension?

____

____

____

____

____

____

____

____

____

____

____

❖ How do you feel about seeking medical advice for
hypertension management? What are your thoughts on
combining herbal remedies with professional guidance for
a holistic approach?

____

____

____

____

____

____

____

❖ Create a personalized action plan for managing hypertension based on the insights gained from this chapter. What specific changes will you implement in your lifestyle, diet, and herbal remedy usage to support your cardiovascular health?

Low Blood Pressure (Hypotension)

This chapter beams light on one of the most neglected conditions known as low blood pressure or hypotension. It simply refers to when the blood pressure is lower than normal at 110/70 mmHg. Hypotension is notably prevalent in adults, which also indicates the body9s need for quality nourishment, rest and vitality.

More so, this chapter explores the root causes of hypotension, emphasizing the importance of addressing inadequate nutrition, lack of rest, insufficient exercise, and underlying health conditions leading to reduced vitality.

Natural remedies for hypotension involve the use of herbs such as hyssop, golden seal, vervain, prickly ash, blue cohosh, gentian, wood betony, burnet, and skullcap. Combining a small amount of red pepper with these herbs enhances their vitality-boosting properties. The chapter provides a simple method for preparing an herbal tea using these herbs to support individuals with low blood pressure.

Diet plays a pivotal role in managing hypotension, with a focus on nourishing foods rich in potassium, including potassium broth, mashed potatoes, baked potatoes (with skin), soybean milk, soy cottage cheese, leafy vegetables, and various other vegetables. The chapter recommends avoiding de-vitaminized or stimulating foods and opting for digestion-friendly options such as peppermint or spearmint tea. Minimizing liquid intake during meals is advised to prevent digestion issues.

Regular outdoor exercise is highlighted as essential for normalizing blood pressure. The chapter introduces Echinacea, known for its blood-toning properties, as a supplementary measure in capsule form.

Reflections and exercises:

❖ Reflect on your awareness of low blood pressure. Were you familiar with the concept, and how do you perceive its significance in comparison to high blood pressure?

____
____
____
____
____
____
____
____
____
____
____
____
____
____
____
____
____
____
____
____
____
____
____
____

❖ Explore potential root causes of hypotension in your life, considering factors such as nutrition, rest, exercise, and underlying health conditions. How might addressing these factors positively impact your overall vitality?

____

____

____

____

____

____

____

____

____

____

____

____

____

____

____

____

____

____

____

____

____

____

____

____

❖   Research and list the herbs mentioned for managing low blood pressure, such as hyssop, golden seal, and blue cohosh. Which of these herbs resonates with you, and how might you incorporate them into your daily routine?

____

____

____

____

____

____

____

____

____

____

____

____

____

____

____

____

____

____

____

____

❖   Experiment with creating the herbal tea blend mentioned in the chapter. How does incorporating this herbal potion into your daily routine impact your energy levels and well-being?

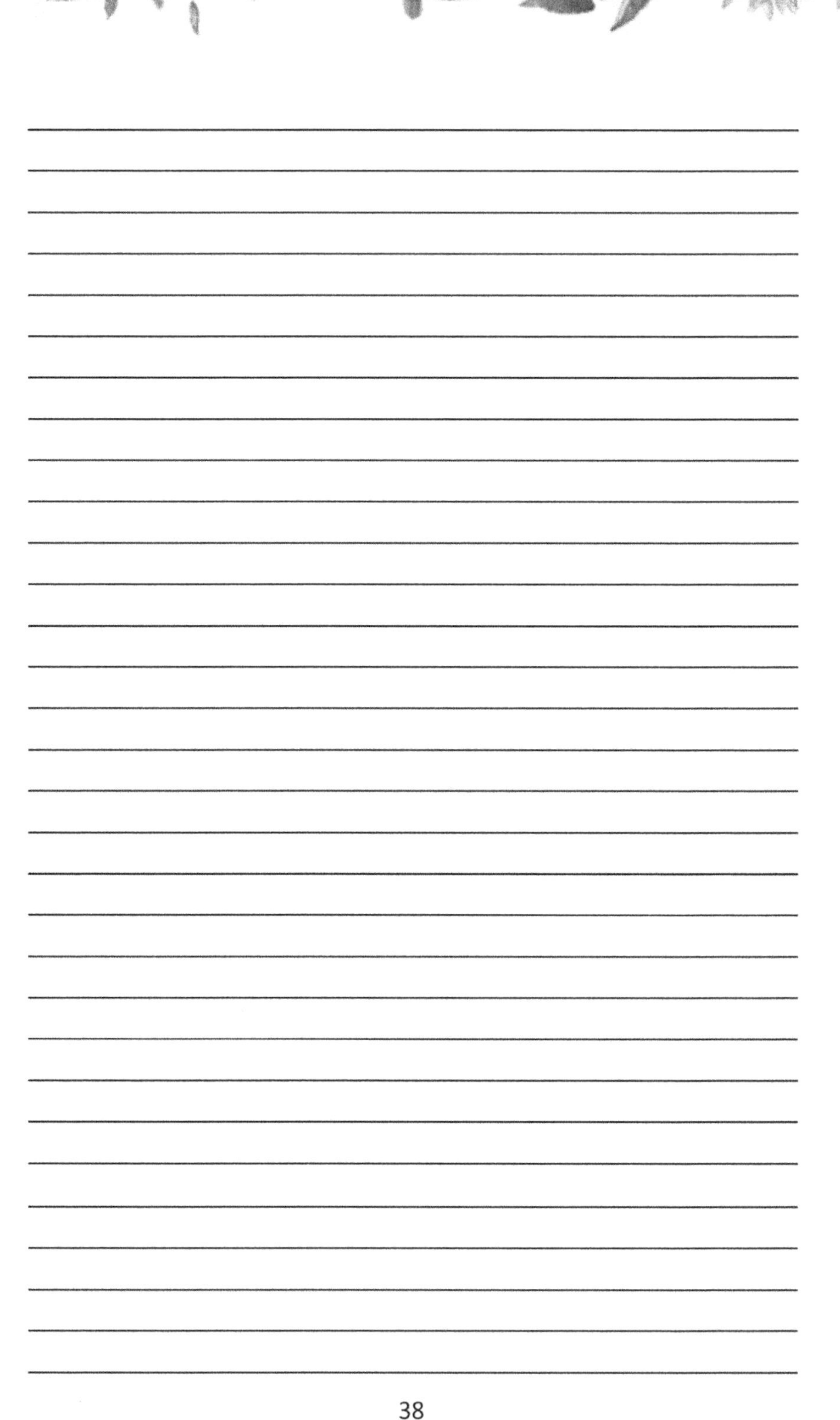

❖ Evaluate your current diet and identify nourishing foods rich in potassium. How can you modify your diet to include these foods and support your body's nutritional needs?

____

____

____

____

____

____

____

____

____

____

____

____

____

____

____

____

____

____

____

____

____

____

____

____

____

❖ Consider the importance of avoiding de-vitaminized or stimulating foods and opting for digestion-friendly options. How can these dietary changes contribute to managing low blood pressure in your daily life?

____

____

____

____

____

____

____

____

____

____

____

____

____

____

❖ Reflect on your current exercise routine. How can you incorporate more outdoor exercise into your lifestyle to support the normalization of blood pressure?

____

____

____

____

____

____

____

____

____

____

____

____

____

____

❖ Research the blood-toning properties of Echinacea. Would you consider incorporating Echinacea supplements into your routine? Why or why not?

____

____

____

____

____

____

____

____

____

____

____

❖ Compare and contrast the management approaches for high blood pressure and low blood pressure discussed in previous chapters. How do these approaches differ, and what common principles can be applied to support overall cardiovascular health?

❖ Develop a personalized action plan for managing hypotension based on the insights gained from this chapter. What specific changes will you implement in your lifestyle, diet, and herbal remedy usage to support your cardiovascular health and vitality?

Acute Myocardial Infarction (Heart Attack)

This chapter delves into acute myocardial infarction, commonly known as a heart attack, a critical medical condition where blood flow to a part of the heart is obstructed, leading to damage or death of the heart muscle. The primary cause is often the buildup of plaque, composed of fat, cholesterol, and cellular waste, in the coronary arteries, resulting in narrowed arteries and reduced blood flow, eventually triggering a heart attack. Key risk factors include coronary artery disease, smoking, high blood pressure, high cholesterol, obesity, sedentary lifestyle, diabetes, poor diet, stress, excessive alcohol consumption, genetics, and age.

While immediate medical attention is crucial in the event of a heart attack, the chapter explores how certain herbs and natural supplements can support heart health and potentially reduce the risk of heart issues. Herbs like hawthorn, garlic, and turmeric are highlighted for their cardiovascular benefits, such as improving blood flow, reducing blood pressure, and enhancing heart functioning.

Reflections and exercises:

- ❖ Reflect on your understanding of acute myocardial infarction (heart attack) before reading this chapter. What new insights or information did you gain regarding the causes and risk factors associated with heart attacks?

____

____

❖ Explore the risk factors mentioned in the chapter for heart attacks, such as smoking, high blood pressure, and poor diet. How do these factors align with your current lifestyle, and what steps can you take to mitigate potential risks?

❖ Research and list the cardiovascular benefits of hawthorn, garlic, and turmeric. Which of these herbs resonates with you, and how might you incorporate them into your daily routine for heart health?

❖ Experiment with preparing one of the herbal potions
mentioned, such as the hawthorn tincture, garlic infusion,
or turmeric tea. How does integrating these natural
remedies into your daily routine impact your overall well-
being?

____

____

____

____

____

____

____

____

____

____

____

____

____

____

____

____

____

____

____

❖ Reflect on the importance of immediate medical attention in the event of a heart attack. Do you have knowledge of emergency response procedures? How can you ensure you and those around you are well-informed and prepared for such situations?

Angina Pectoris

This chapter explores Angina Pectoris, commonly known as angina, a condition characterized by chest pain or discomfort arising from insufficient blood flow to the heart muscle, often due to narrowing or blockage in the coronary arteries. The root cause of angina is coronary artery disease (CAD), primarily associated with risk factors such as high cholesterol, hypertension, smoking, diabetes, sedentary lifestyle, unhealthy eating habits, and stress. The chapter emphasizes the role of traditional herbal remedies in managing angina and improving heart health, featuring herbs like hawthorn berry, garlic, ginkgo biloba, and motherwort.

Hawthorn berry is recognized for its cardiovascular benefits, dilating blood vessels and enhancing blood flow to the heart. Garlic reduces cholesterol levels and blood pressure, mitigating the risk of plaque buildup. Ginkgo biloba improves circulation and is beneficial in coronary artery disease, while motherwort acts as a heart tonic, reducing palpitations and enhancing heart function.

The chapter concludes with recipes for herbal potions using these herbs, such as Hawthorn Berry Tincture, Garlic Infusion, Ginkgo Biloba Tea, and Motherwort Tea, providing practical guidance on their preparation and usage.

Reflections and exercises:

- ❖ Reflect on your understanding of angina pectoris before reading this chapter. How has your perception of angina evolved, and what key factors contribute to this cardiovascular condition?

____

____

____

____

____

____

____

____

____

____

____

____

____

____

____

____

____

____

❖ Examine the risk factors associated with angina, as mentioned in the chapter. Which of these factors align with your current lifestyle, and how can you modify your habits to reduce the risk of developing angina?

____

____

____

____

____

____

____

____

❖ Research the cardiovascular benefits of hawthorn berry, garlic, ginkgo biloba, and motherwort. How do these herbs contribute to heart health, and which one resonates with you the most?

❖ Experiment with preparing one of the herbal potions mentioned, such as the Hawthorn Berry Tincture or Garlic Infusion. How does incorporating these natural remedies into your routine impact your overall well-being?

❖ Explore stress management techniques to reduce emotional triggers for angina episodes. How can incorporating practices like mindfulness, meditation, or relaxation exercises contribute to managing stress and preventing angina attacks

Hyperlipidemia

This chapter explores hyperlipidemia, a condition characterized by elevated levels of lipids (fats) in the bloodstream, including cholesterol and triglycerides. Hyperlipidemia often has a multifaceted origin, involving genetic predispositions and lifestyle factors. While genetic factors may contribute, for most individuals, dietary and lifestyle choices play a significant role. The condition is identified as a major risk factor for cardiovascular diseases, such as heart attacks and strokes.

The primary causes of hyperlipidemia are rooted in diet and lifestyle choices. Diets high in saturated fats, trans fats, and cholesterol, along with sedentary lifestyles, obesity, excessive alcohol consumption, and smoking, contribute to elevated lipid levels. Additionally, underlying health conditions like diabetes and thyroid disorders can exacerbate or trigger hyperlipidemia.

The chapter introduces traditional herbal remedies for managing hyperlipidemia, featuring herbs like garlic, guggul, red yeast rice, artichoke leaf, and green tea. These herbs are known for their cholesterol-lowering properties and their ability to address lipid levels in the body.

Herbal potions for hyperlipidemia include the Garlic Potion, Guggul Potion, Red Yeast Rice Brew, Artichoke Leaf Tea, and Green Tea, each offering a natural approach to lipid management.

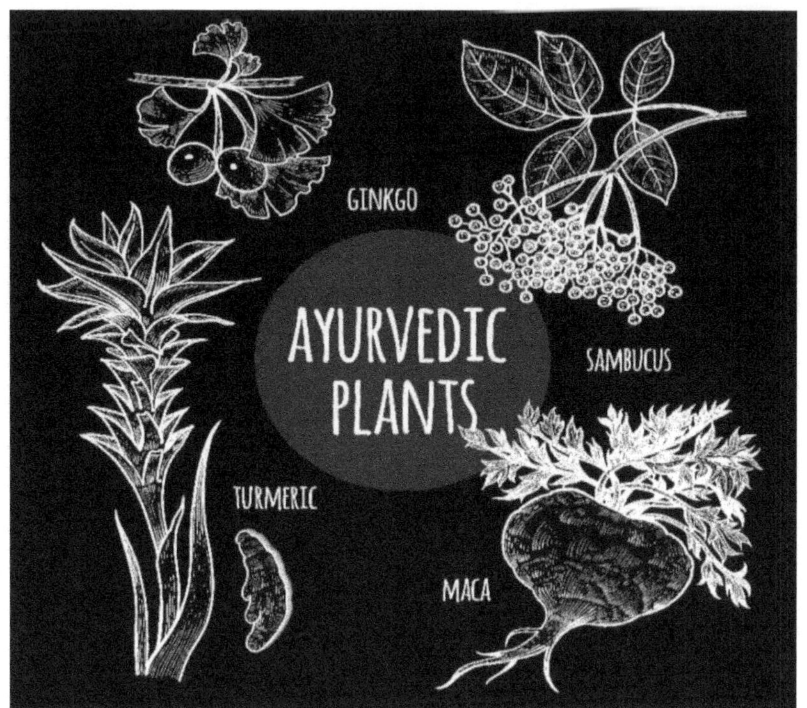

Reflections and exercises:

- ❖ This chapter explores Reflect on your knowledge of hyperlipidemia before reading this chapter. What new insights or information have you gained regarding the causes and risks associated with elevated lipid levels?

____

____

____

____

❖ Evaluate your current dietary and lifestyle choices in relation to the causes of hyperlipidemia mentioned in the chapter. How might modifications to your diet and habits contribute to the management of lipid levels in your body?

____

____

____

____

❖ Research the cholesterol-lowering properties of garlic,
   guggul, red yeast rice, artichoke leaf, and green tea. Which
   of these herbs resonates with you, and how could you
   incorporate it into your daily routine?

____

____

____

____

____

____

____

____

____

____

____

____

____

____

❖ Experiment with preparing one of the herbal potions
mentioned, such as the Garlic Potion or Artichoke Leaf
Tea. How does integrating these natural remedies into your
routine impact your approach to managing hyperlipidemia?

❖ Explore lifestyle changes to complement herbal remedies
for hyperlipidemia. How can incorporating regular
exercise, maintaining a healthy weight, and reducing
alcohol consumption contribute to a holistic approach in
managing lipid levels?

Arrhythmias (many are painless)

This chapter explores arrhythmias, irregular heartbeats characterized by the heart beating too quickly, too slowly, or with an erratic pattern. The root causes of arrhythmias are attributed to disruptions in the electrical impulses that control the heartbeat. When these impulses malfunction, they lead to irregular heartbeats, often felt as fluttering, racing, or slow heartbeats.

Diverse factors contribute to the root causes of arrhythmias, including heart disease, high blood pressure, diabetes, smoking, heavy alcohol use, excessive caffeine consumption, certain medications, and stress. Additionally, electrolyte imbalances in the body can also contribute to the occurrence of arrhythmias, and in some cases, the exact cause remains unknown.

The chapter introduces natural remedies for managing arrhythmias, highlighting herbs with heart-regulating properties. Hawthorn berry is recognized for its ability to improve circulation, regulate heartbeat, and strengthen the heart muscle. Other beneficial herbs include motherwort, known for calming heart palpitations and reducing heart stress, and valerian, appreciated for its relaxing properties.

Herbal potions for arrhythmias include the Hawthorn Berry Tincture, Motherwort Tea, and Valerian Root Infusion, each offering a natural approach to support heart health.

Reflections and exercises:

❖ Reflect on your understanding of arrhythmias before reading this chapter. What aspects of irregular heartbeats were you familiar with, and how has your knowledge evolved?

____

____

____

____

____

____

❖   Evaluate your lifestyle in relation to the root causes of
    arrhythmias mentioned in the chapter. Which factors align
    with your current habits, and how can you modify your
    lifestyle to reduce the risk of experiencing arrhythmias?

____

____

____

____

____

____

____

____

____

____

____

____

____

❖ Research the heart-regulating properties of hawthorn berry, motherwort, and valerian. How might incorporating these herbs into your routine contribute to managing and preventing arrhythmias?

Silent Myocardial Infarction (asymptomatic)

This chapter explores silent myocardial infarction, an asymptomatic heart attack that often goes unnoticed, detected only later through medical imaging or routine electrocardiograms (ECG). Unlike classic heart attacks, the danger of a silent myocardial infarction lies in its ability to go undetected, leaving individuals unaware of the heart damage they have sustained.

The root causes of silent myocardial infarction include high cholesterol levels, hypertension, smoking, diabetes, and a sedentary lifestyle. These factors contribute to the development of atherosclerosis, the primary condition leading to blockages in the arteries.

In addition to previously mentioned remedies like Hawthorn Berry Tincture, Garlic Infusion, and Gingko Biloba Tea, the chapter introduces other herbs to support heart health, including turmeric, ginger, flaxseed, and cayenne pepper. These herbs are known for their anti-inflammatory properties, ability to improve blood circulation, and contribute to overall heart health.

Herbal potions for silent myocardial infarction include Turmeric Tea, Ginger Infusion, Flaxseed Drink, and Cayenne Pepper Tonic, each providing a natural approach to support cardiovascular well-being.

Reflections and exercises:

- ❖ Reflect on your awareness of silent myocardial infarction before reading this chapter. How does the concept of an asymptomatic heart attack impact your understanding of cardiovascular health?

❖ Examine the root causes mentioned in the chapter for silent myocardial infarction. How do these causes align with your current lifestyle, and what steps can you take to modify your habits to reduce the risk of silent heart damage?

❖ Research the heart-supporting properties of turmeric, ginger, flaxseed, and cayenne pepper. How might incorporating these herbs into your routine contribute to reducing the risk of silent myocardial infarction?

Aortic Aneurysm

This chapter delves into aortic aneurysm, a serious condition characterized by an abnormal bulge in the aorta, the body's largest blood vessel supplying blood to the abdomen, pelvis, and legs. Aortic aneurysms can be silent, revealing themselves through symptoms only when they become large or rupture. The potential rupture of an aortic aneurysm can lead to dangerous, sometimes fatal bleeding.

The root causes of aortic aneurysms vary, often including factors such as atherosclerosis (hardening of the arteries), hypertension (high blood pressure), genetic conditions, and lifestyle factors like smoking. Over time, these conditions weaken the arterial wall, contributing to the formation of an aneurysm.

In addition to previously mentioned remedies like Hawthorn Berry Tincture, Garlic Infusion, and Gingko Biloba Tea, the chapter introduces other herbs that may support arterial health and potentially mitigate the risks associated with aortic aneurysm, including turmeric, green tea, and cayenne pepper.

Herbal potions for aortic aneurysm include the Turmeric Potion, Green Tea Brew, and Cayenne Pepper Tonic, offering a natural approach to support arterial health.

Reflections and exercises:

❖ Reflect on your knowledge of aortic aneurysm before reading this chapter. How does understanding the potential risks and causes impact your awareness of cardiovascular health?

____

____

____

❖ Examine the root causes mentioned in the chapter for silent myocardial infarction. How do these causes align with your current lifestyle, and what steps can you take to modify your habits to reduce the risk of silent heart damage?

❖ Research the arterial health benefits of turmeric, green tea, and cayenne pepper. How might incorporating these herbs into your routine contribute to maintaining the health of your blood vessels

❖ Consider the potential silent nature of aortic aneurysms. How can regular check-ups and medical imaging contribute to the early detection and prevention of complications associated with aortic aneurysms?

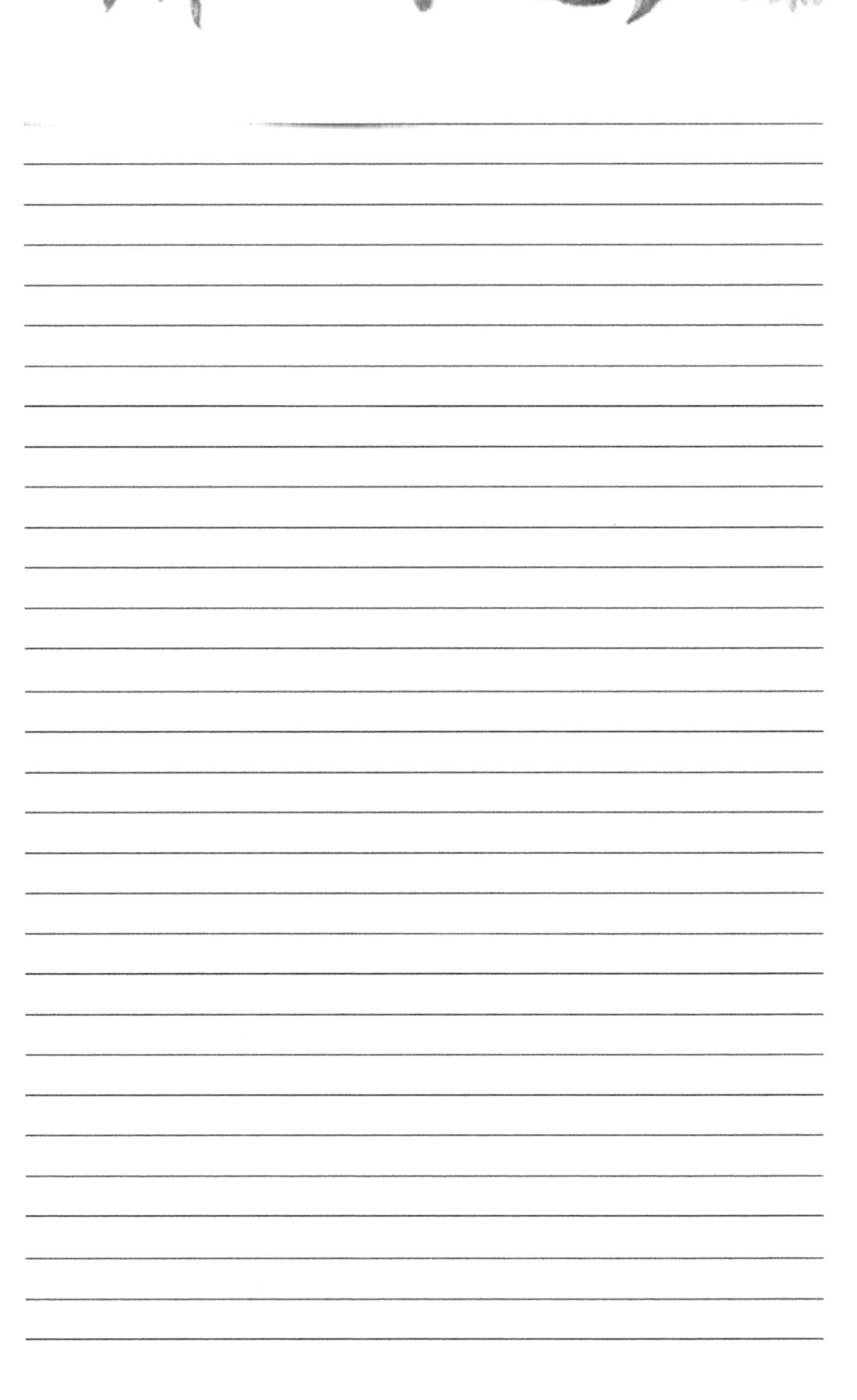

6. Peripheral Artery Disease (PAD)

This chapter explores Peripheral Arterial Disease (PAD), a condition originating from the buildup of fatty deposits in the arteries, primarily affecting those in the legs. PAD restricts blood flow, leading to symptoms such as leg pain when walking (claudication), numbness, or weakness in the legs.

The root cause of PAD is often atherosclerosis, a process where arteries harden and narrow due to the accumulation of plaques. Lifestyle factors such as smoking, high cholesterol, high blood pressure, and diabetes contribute to the development of PAD.

In addition to previously mentioned remedies like Hawthorn Berry Tincture, Garlic Infusion, and Gingko Biloba Tea, the chapter introduces other herbs that may be effective in managing PAD, including Horse Chestnut Extract, Turmeric, and Ginger. These herbs are known for their abilities to improve vascular health, reduce inflammation, and enhance blood circulation.

Herbal potions for PAD include the Horse Chestnut Extract Potion, Turmeric Potion, and Ginger Potion, offering a natural and complementary approach to managing PAD alongside lifestyle changes and medical treatments.

Reflections and exercises:

- ❖ Reflect on your knowledge of Peripheral Arterial Disease (PAD) before reading this chapter. How do the symptoms described align with or differ from your previous understanding of arterial health?

____

____

❖ Examine the root causes mentioned in the chapter for PAD. How do these causes align with your current lifestyle, and what modifications can you make to reduce the risk of developing PAD?

____

____

____

____

____

____

____

____

____

____

❖ Research the vascular health benefits of Horse Chestnut Extract, Turmeric, and Ginger. How might incorporating these herbs into your routine contribute to managing symptoms of PAD and improving overall arterial health?

____

____

____

____

____

____

____

____

____

____

____

____

____

❖ Consider the importance of standardized formulations when using herbal remedies for PAD, as mentioned for Horse Chestnut Extract. How can individuals ensure the safety and effectiveness of herbal treatments, and what resources can they consult for guidance?

Hemorrhage

This chapter takes a look at hemorrhages in various forms, such as bleeding from the lungs, uterus, bowels, and nose. Traditional remedies suggest specific herbs for each type, focusing on their astringent properties to constrict blood vessels and reduce bleeding. Herbs like Bayberry Bark, Bistort Root, Red Raspberry Leaves, White Oak Bark, Witch Hazel Bark, Wild Alum Root, Shepherd's Purse, Sumac, Golden Seal, and Blackberry Leaves are celebrated for their effectiveness in managing hemorrhages.

Interestingly, the root cause of hemorrhages generally involves the rupture or weakness of blood vessels. While herbal remedies are often effective, persistent bleeding should be evaluated by a physician as it may indicate serious conditions like cancer.

Herbal potions for lung and uterine hemorrhages involve steeping bayberry bark or bistort root in boiling water, while bowel hemorrhages can be addressed with enemas using wild alum root, white oak bark, or red raspberry tea. Nosebleeds may be managed with a goldenseal tea or a combination of wild alum root, blackberry leaves, witch hazel leaves, and white oak bark.

❖ Reflect on your knowledge of hemorrhages before reading this chapter. How has your understanding of herbal remedies for different types of bleeding evolved?

____

____

____

❖ Evaluate the root causes mentioned in the chapter for hemorrhages. How do these causes align with your current knowledge, and what steps can you take to minimize the risk of hemorrhages?

____

____

____

____

____

____

____

____

____

____

____

____

____

____

____

____

____

❖ Research the astringent and healing properties of herbs
mentioned for managing hemorrhages. How can these
properties contribute to reducing bleeding and promoting
recovery?

____

____

____

____

____

____

❖ Consider the importance of seeking medical evaluation for persistent bleeding, as mentioned in the chapter. How can individuals strike a balance between herbal remedies and professional medical advice in managing hemorrhages?

7. **Deep Vein Thrombosis**

This chapter delves into the often-underdiscussed health issue of Deep Vein Thrombosis (DVT), where blood clots form deep within veins, particularly in the legs. The disruption of blood flow can lead to swelling, pain, and various complications. DVT is linked to factors such as prolonged inactivity, certain medications, smoking, obesity, and heart disease.

The chapter introduces herbal remedies as guardians against DVT, featuring lesser-known yet potent allies. Ginkgo Biloba, known for improving blood circulation and reducing clot formation; Hawthorn berries, celebrated for strengthening blood vessels; and Horse Chestnut, valued for reducing swelling and improving blood flow.

Herbal potions for DVT include Ginkgo Biloba Tea, Hawthorn Berry Tonic, and Horse Chestnut Salve. These remedies offer a natural approach to support cardiovascular health and reduce the risk of blood clot formation.

Reflections and exercises:

- ❖ Reflect on your understanding of Deep Vein Thrombosis (DVT) before reading this chapter. How has your perception of this health issue evolved, and what aspects surprised you?

____

____

____

❖ Explore the root causes mentioned in the chapter for DVT. How do these causes align with potential lifestyle factors, and what adjustments can you make to reduce the risk of DVT?

❖ Research the historical uses and health benefits of Ginkgo Biloba, Hawthorn berries, and Horse Chestnut. How do these herbal allies contribute to cardiovascular health, and what other lifestyle habits complement their effects?

____

____

____

____

____

____

____

____

____

____

____

____

❖ Consider the herbal potions provided in the chapter. How can the brewing and application of these remedies be incorporated into a daily routine to support overall vascular health and prevent DVT?

____

____

____

____

____

____

____

Varicose Veins

This chapter briefly explores varicose veins, which result from prolonged standing, sluggish circulation, pregnancy, or inherited factors, leading to enlarged and knotted veins in the legs, causing pain and potential skin ulcers. The management of varicose veins involves a nourishing diet, regular bowel movements, cold baths, special stockings, and topical applications like white oak bark tea for relief. Severe cases may benefit from an herbal blend of goldenseal, myrrh, hyssop, white cherry bark, and yellow dock root.

The root causes of varicose veins include prolonged standing, poor circulation, pregnancy, and genetic factors, leading to the enlargement and twisting of veins.

Recommended herbal remedies for varicose veins include White Oak Bark, Witch Hazel, Bayberry Bark, Wild Alum Root, and Burnet. Herbal potions involve a Golden Seal and Myrrh Tea for internal use and a mix of Hyssop, White Cherry Bark, and Yellow Dock Root for specific dosage throughout the day. External applications involve a strong tea of white oak bark applied to affected limbs.

Reflections and exercises:

❖ How has your understanding of the causes and management of varicose veins evolved after reading this chapter?

❖ Examine the root causes outlined in the chapter for varicose veins. How do these factors align with potential aspects of your lifestyle, and what changes can you make to minimize the risk of developing varicose veins?

____
____
____
____
____
____
____
____
____
____
____
____
____
____

❖ Investigate the properties and benefits of the recommended herbs for varicose veins, including White Oak Bark, Witch Hazel, Bayberry Bark, Wild Alum Root, and Burnet. In what ways do these herbs contribute to alleviating symptoms and promoting vascular health?

____
____
____
____
____

____

____

____

____

____

____

____

____

____

❖ Deliberate on the herbal potions provided in the chapter. How can you integrate the brewing and consumption of these remedies into your daily routine to support the management of varicose veins effectively?

____

____

____

____

____

____

____

____

____

____

____

____

8. PULMONARY EMBOLISM (PE)

Pulmonary embolism (PE) poses a serious threat as blood clots, often originating in the veins of the legs or pelvis, can travel to the lungs, causing life-threatening blockages. The primary cause, deep vein thrombosis (DVT), involves clots forming in deeper veins. Herbal remedies, including Pleurisy Root, Lobelia, Beth Root, Colombo, and Horehound, are traditionally believed to offer relief and support respiratory health.

Reflections and exercises:

❖ Explore the root causes of pulmonary embolism outlined in the chapter. How do factors like prolonged immobility and genetic predispositions contribute to the development of deep vein thrombosis?

❖ Investigate the properties of the recommended herbs for pulmonary embolism. How can Pleurisy Root, Lobelia, Beth Root, Colombo, and Horehound collectively contribute to respiratory health and blood circulation?

❖ Discuss the herbal potions suggested in the chapter. How can incorporating Pleurisy Root tea, Lobelia tincture, Beth Root brew, Colombo infusion, and Horehound syrup into a routine potentially aid in managing pulmonary embolism?

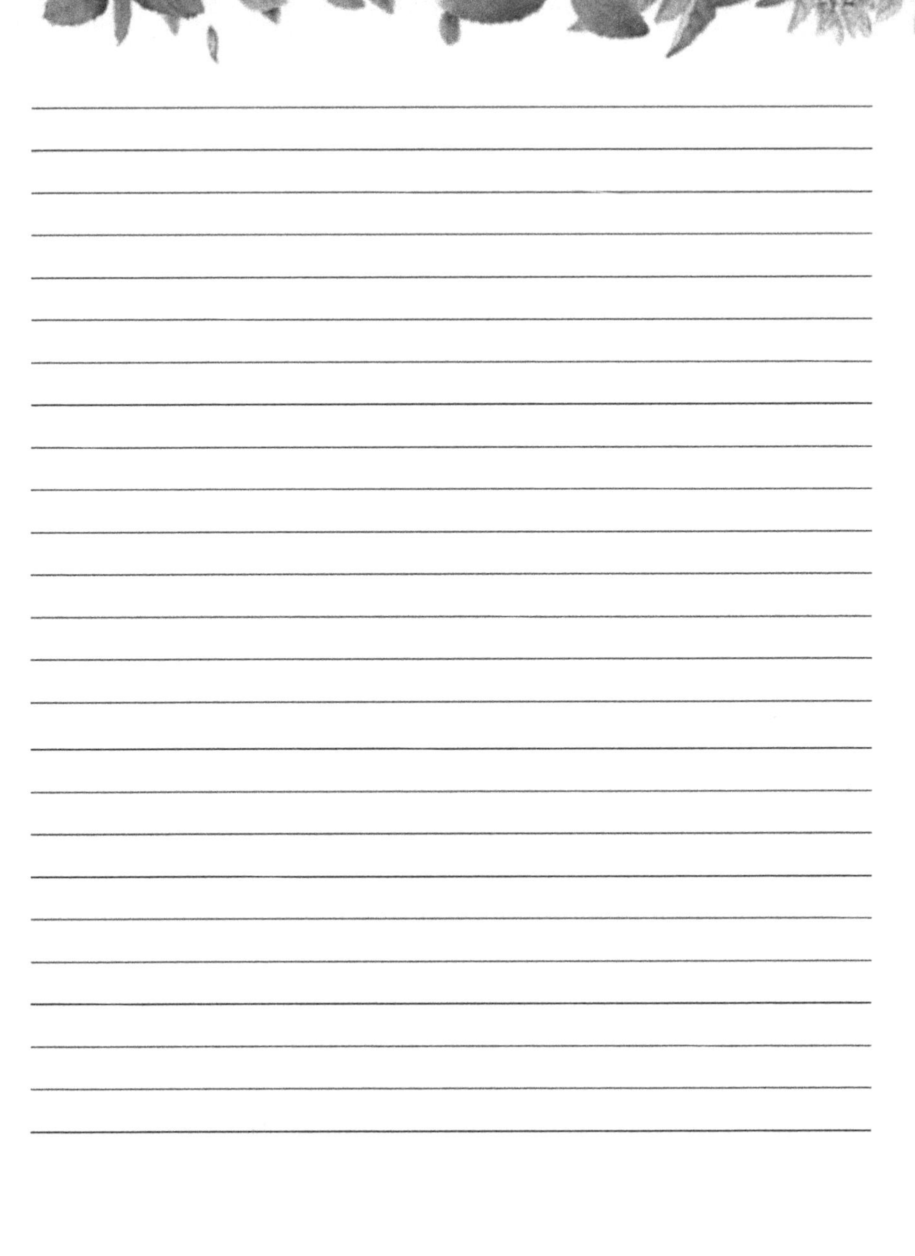

Nosebleeds, commonly caused by factors such as nasal injury, environmental exposure, or blood abnormalities, can benefit from herbal remedies. Goldenseal, wild alum root, white oak bark, bayberry bark, and ephedra vulgaris are recognized for their healing properties and effectiveness in addressing nosebleeds, sinus issues, and colds.

Reflections and exercises:

- ❖ Examine the root cause of nosebleeds as discussed in the chapter. How do acute stress on nasal blood vessels contribute to this common occurrence, and what are the potential triggers?

____

____

____

____

____

____

____

____

____

____

- ❖ Explore the versatility of the recommended herbs. How can goldenseal, wild alum root, white oak bark, bayberry bark, and ephedra vulgaris provide relief not only for nosebleeds but also for sinus issues and colds?

____

____

❖ Deliberate on the herbal potions outlined. How can the Golden Seal solution, a blend of Wild Alum Root, White Oak Bark, or Bayberry Bark, and Ephedra Vulgaris infusion be prepared and effectively used for managing nosebleeds?

❖ Consider the historical use of herbal remedies for nosebleeds. How have these remedies been traditionally employed across cultures, and what insights can be gained from their longstanding efficacy?

____
____
____
____
____
____
____
____
____
____
____
____
____
____

9. Sinus Difficulties

Sinus difficulties are often associated with infections like the common cold or flu. They can result from blockage and infection in the sinuses. Frequent underwater activities and poor lifestyle choices can contribute to these issues, manifesting symptoms such as severe pain, eye aches, nasal discharge, headaches, and fever resembling hay fever symptoms. The primary cause is the blockage of channels connecting sinuses to the nasal cavity, commonly due to infections and lifestyle factors. A holistic approach involving diet and herbal remedies, despite being downplayed by pharmaceutical companies, is recommended for managing sinus troubles.

Reflections and exercises:

❖ What are the contributing factors to sinus difficulties outlined in the chapter? Explain how infections in the nose and throat, along with lifestyle choices, play a role in the blockage of sinus channels.

____
____
____
____
____
____
____
____
____
____
____
____
____
____
____
____
____
____
____

❖ Discuss the recommended natural remedies for addressing sinus difficulties. How does a 4-5 day fruit juice fast,

followed by a vegetable-rich diet, aid in managing sinus
issues, and what is the reasoning behind these dietary
recommendations?

____

____

____

____

____

____

____

____

____

____

____

____

____

____

____

____

____

____

____

____

❖ Evaluate the effectiveness of cold and hot applications for
sinus relief. Elaborate on the benefits of alternating
between cold and hot compresses on the sinuses and why
customization based on individual comfort is emphasized.

❖ What are the early non-specific symptoms of poliomyelitis discussed in this chapter?

____

____

____

____

____

____

____

____

____

____

____

____

____

____

____

____

____

____

❖ Name three herbs mentioned as effective in supporting the treatment of polio symptoms through herbal remedies.

____

____

____

contribute to cleansing and healing the nasal passages, and what is the suggested application method?

____

____

____

____

____

____

____

____

____

____

____

____

____

____

____

____

____

____

____

____

____

____

____

____

Pericarditis

Pericarditis is characterized by inflammation of the pericardium, the membrane surrounding the heart. The root causes vary, including infectious factors (viral, bacterial, fungal), non-infectious factors (autoimmune disorders, post-heart attack syndrome, trauma), and other causes like kidney failure, medications, radiation therapy, and cancer. A herbal potion is suggested for symptom relief, emphasizing anti-inflammatory and heart-healthy herbs like garlic, ginger, turmeric, and hawthorn. Caution is advised, and consultation with a healthcare provider is crucial before starting any new treatment.

Reflections and exercises:

❖ What are the diverse root causes of pericarditis, and how do infectious, non-infectious, and other factors contribute to the development of this medical condition?

____
____
____
____
____
____
____
____
____

❖ Explain the rationale behind using herbs like garlic, ginger, turmeric, and hawthorn in the herbal potion for pericarditis. How do these herbs address inflammation and support heart health?

❖ Outline the step-by-step process for preparing the herbal potion. What considerations should be taken into account, such as dosage and potential sweetening with honey?

❖ Discuss the importance of consulting with a healthcare provider before using the herbal remedy for pericarditis. Why is this precaution necessary, especially for individuals with underlying health conditions or those taking medications?

PART IV: NEUROLOGICAL DISORDER

The upcoming chapters delve into the potential effectiveness of herbs in managing various neurological disorders. Neurological conditions can significantly impact an individual's quality of life, often requiring complex and multifaceted treatment approaches. In these chapters, the author explore the traditional uses of herbs and natural remedies that have been suggested to provide relief for conditions affecting the nervous system. While these herbal approaches are discussed, it's crucial to note that they should be considered as complementary strategies, and consultation with healthcare professionals remains essential for comprehensive care. Let's embark on a journey to understand how certain herbs may offer support and relief in the realm of neurological health.

10. Migraines, Cluster Headaches

This chapter explores the debilitating nature of migraines and cluster headaches, emphasizing the diverse root causes that often overlap. Dental infections, urinary tract infections, bowel issues, and the presence of a wormlet named Strongyloides are highlighted as contributors.

Food allergies, especially reactions to dairy, eggs, citrus, and salty foods, can further exacerbate migraine symptoms. The chapter proposes a sustainable approach using herbal remedies to target root causes directly, including parasite cleanses, dental infection remedies, bowel cleansing, and liver cleanses.

Reflections and exercises:

❖ What are some of the diverse root causes of migraines and cluster headaches discussed in this chapter?

____

____

____

____

____

____

____

____

____

____

____

____

____

____

❖ How can herbal remedies contribute to addressing Strongyloides-related migraines? Provide an example of an herbal remedy mentioned.

❖ Why is it mentioned that avoiding certain trigger foods long-term is challenging, and what alternative approach is suggested?

❖ Explain the steps involved in making the herbal potion for dental infections using white iodine or Lugol's solution.

11. Infant Paralysis (Polio Myletis)

Infantile paralysis, also known as poliomyelitis, is a viral disease primarily spread through human contact and affecting various bodily systems. The early symptoms include non-specific indicators like fever, fatigue, muscle aches, and gastrointestinal issues, with more severe manifestations leading to muscle weakness and paralysis.

Despite the success of vaccination programs, traditional herbal remedies have demonstrated promising results in managing polio symptoms.

❖ What are the early non-specific symptoms of poliomyelitis discussed in this chapter?

____

____

____

____

____

____

____

____

____

____

____

____

____

____

____

____

____

❖ Name three herbs mentioned as effective in supporting the treatment of polio symptoms through herbal remedies.

____

____

____

❖ How can a herbal tea be prepared using valerian, catnip, and calamus root for managing infantile paralysis?

____

____

____

____

____

____

❖ Explain the suggested dosage and administration of the herbal tea for children, and why is it recommended to be sweetened with honey or malt sugar?

____

____

____

____

____

____

____

____

____

____

____

____

____

12.   Sciatica

This chapter explores sciatica, a condition associated with problems related to the sciatic nerve, characterized by pain radiating along the nerve's path from the lower back through the buttocks and down the legs.

Some of the root causes of sciatica include issues like lumbar spinal stenosis, degenerative disc disease, herniated disc, piriformis syndrome, pregnancy, and muscle spasms. Herbal remedies, featuring Rue, Wintergreen, Broom, Burdock, and Tansy, are discussed for their potential anti-inflammatory and analgesic properties.

Reflections and exercises:

❖ What are the common sources of irritation leading to sciatica, as discussed in this chapter?

____

____

____

____

____

____

____

____

____

____

____

____

____

____

❖ Name three herbs mentioned for their potential to relieve sciatica pain and their believed properties.

❖ Outline the general steps for creating an herbal potion for sciatica relief, emphasizing key considerations.

❖ How can the dosage of the herbal potion vary, and why is it essential to consider individual health conditions?

13. Narcolepsy

This chapter briefly delves into narcolepsy, a chronic neurological disorder affecting sleep-wake cycles due to abnormal brain functioning. The root cause involves factors like genetic predisposition and the loss of hypocretin-producing brain cells, potentially triggered by an autoimmune response.

While there is no known cure for narcolepsy, herbal remedies like Valerian Root, Chamomile, Lemon Balm, St. John9s Wort, and Passionflower are discussed for managing symptoms. A simple herbal potion using chamomile and lemon balm is provided, emphasizing the need for consultation with healthcare providers before herbal treatment.

Reflections and exercises:

❖ Explain the origin of the term "narcolepsy" and its connection to the disorder's characteristics.

____

____

____

____

____

____

❖ What factors contribute to the root cause of narcolepsy, as mentioned in the chapter?

❖ List three herbs traditionally used for managing sleep disorders, and briefly describe their potential effects.

- ❖ Provide a step-by-step guide to preparing the herbal potion mentioned in the chapter for aiding sleep in individuals with narcolepsy.

21. Headaches

This chapter carefully explores headaches, categorizing them into sick headaches, bilious headaches, and nervous (tension) headaches, each with distinct root causes. It emphasizes the effectiveness of natural herbal remedies in treating headaches despite pharmaceutical industry biases.

Remedies include hot footbaths, cold compresses, and herbal teas for sick headaches, dietary moderation and enemas for bilious headaches, and rest, herbal teas, and enemas for nervous headaches. Herbal potions involve teas, footbaths, liniments, and enemas using various herbs, offering a holistic approach to headache relief.

Reflections and exercises:

❖ What are the root causes of sick headaches, bilious headaches, and nervous (tension) headaches as discussed in the chapter?

____
____
____
____
____
____
____
____
____
____

❖ Provide three herbal remedies suggested for treating sick headaches and briefly explain their benefits.

❖ Explain the dietary and treatment recommendations for addressing bilious headaches according to the chapter.

❖ Describe the holistic approach to managing nervous headaches, including herbal teas, liniments, and enemas mentioned in the chapter.

❖ Sleep Apnea

This chapter beams light on sleep apnea, identifying its root causes as environmental toxins, allergies, and infections leading to throat swelling and airway restriction. The impact of environmental factors, allergic reactions, and infections, along with the role of persistent metals in the mouth, is discussed.

This chapter emphasizes a holistic approach to managing sleep apnea, incorporating herbs such as turmeric, echinacea, and licorice root known for their anti-inflammatory, immune-boosting, and soothing properties.

Herbal potions, including turmeric tea, echinacea tincture, and licorice root tea, are provided as natural remedies for reducing throat swelling and supporting immunity.

Reflections and exercises:

❖ What are the primary root causes of sleep apnea discussed in the chapter, and how do they contribute to the condition?

____

____

____

____

____

____

____

____

____

____

____

____

____

____

❖ Explain the environmental factors mentioned in the chapter that can lead to throat swelling and contribute to sleep apnea.

❖ Describe the holistic approach suggested in the chapter for managing sleep apnea, including the herbs recommended and their properties..

❖ Provide the step-by-step instructions for making turmeric tea, echinacea tincture, and licorice root tea as mentioned in the chapter.

____

____

____

____

____

____

____

____

____

____

____

____

❖ Vertigo

Vertigo is a condition characterized by a spinning or swaying sensation when a person is not moving. It can range from a minor annoyance to a debilitating condition. The root causes of vertigo often involve issues with the inner ear, such as Benign Paroxysmal Positional Vertigo (BPPV), Meniere's Disease, or Vestibular Neuritis.

Various herbal remedies, including ginger, Ginkgo Biloba, and peppermint, are believed to alleviate vertigo symptoms. A simple ginger tea recipe is provided as a natural remedy.

Reflections and exercises:

❖ What is the common name for the sensation of spinning or swaying associated with vertigo, and how is it often described?

❖ Explain the root causes of vertigo and provide brief descriptions of at least two common conditions associated with it.

❖ Why is it important to consult with a healthcare professional before trying herbal remedies for vertigo, and what are three herbal remedies mentioned in the chapter?

____

____

____

____

____

____

____

____

❖ Provide a step-by-step guide to preparing the ginger tea mentioned as a natural remedy for vertigo, and discuss how often it can be consumed according to the chapter.

____

____

____

____

____

____

____

____

____

____

❖ Bell9s Palsy

Palsy is known to often result from nerve fatigue or injury influenced by dietary factors, and leads to symptoms like limb trembling. Treatment involves eliminating certain foods and adopting an elimination diet. While permanent nerve damage may hinder complete recovery, various methods like hot and cold applications, massages, and herbal remedies can provide relief.

Bell's palsy, causing sudden facial muscle paralysis, usually heals in weeks, while cerebral palsy, a more severe form, is related to brain damage and requires long-term management, including speech therapy and muscle training. The root cause of palsy is nerve damage, worsened by dietary factors, with cerebral palsy involving complex issues like oxygen deprivation or infections during childbirth.

Reflections and exercises:

❖ What dietary choices are mentioned in the chapter as potential contributors to palsy, and how do these impact nerve health?

❖ Explain the difference between Bell's palsy and cerebral palsy, including their symptoms and usual recovery timelines.

❖ What are some suggested methods for managing and alleviating the symptoms of palsy, particularly in its less severe forms?

❖ Provide a step-by-step guide to preparing the Prickly Ash
  and Lobelia Potion mentioned as a natural remedy for
  palsy, and discuss the potential benefits of each ingredient
  in the mixture.

❖ Neuralgia

Neuralgia is a condition characterized by nerve irritation, often
triggered by factors such as exposure to dampness, cold, dental

decay, improper diets, eyestrain, and infections around the nose. The primary symptom is localized pain along the affected nerve, sometimes accompanied by muscle weakness, paralysis, or reduced skin sensation.

Natural remedies for neuralgia involve a blend of herbs known for their nerve-soothing properties, including Valerian, Origanum, Skullcap, Queen of the Meadow, Nettle, Poplar bark, Peppermint, Solomon's Seal, Hops, Lady's Slipper, Twinleaf, Motherwort, and Wood Betony. A herbal potion can be prepared by steeping these herbs in boiling water and consuming the tea or using it as a hot fomentation for the affected area. Hot and cold compresses, as well as herbal liniments, can provide relief, and maintaining a nourishing diet with sufficient vitamin E is essential for managing neuralgia.

Reflections and exercises:

❖ What are some contributing factors to neuralgia mentioned in the chapter, and how do they affect the development of this condition?

____

____

❖ Name at least six herbs recommended for alleviating
neuralgia symptoms and briefly explain their nerve-
soothing properties.

____
____
____
____
____
____
____
____
____
____
____
____
____
____

❖ Provide a step-by-step guide to preparing the herbal potion
for neuralgia mentioned in the chapter, and explain how it
can be used for relief.

____
____
____
____
____

❖ Discuss the additional remedies mentioned for neuralgia, such as hot and cold compresses, herbal liniments, and immersing the opposite hand and arm in hot water, and explain how each may contribute to alleviating neuralgia discomfort.

❖ Azheimer9s Disease and Dementia

Alzheimer's disease and Dementia, often associated with aging, are linked to a decline in the liver's ability to detoxify toxins, leading to symptoms like memory loss and disorientation. Combatting these symptoms involves reducing exposure to common toxins through lifestyle changes, particularly in diet and environment.

The root cause of these symptoms in aging individuals lies in the decreased efficiency of the liver in detoxifying harmful substances. Natural remedies include herbs like milk thistle, dandelion root, and turmeric, known for their liver-supporting and detoxification properties. Herbal potions, such as Milk Thistle Tea, Dandelion Root Tea, and Turmeric Tea, can be prepared and consumed regularly to enhance liver function and aid detoxification.

Reflections and exercises:

❖ Explain the connection between mental deterioration in the elderly, Alzheimer's disease, and Dementia, and the role of the liver in this context.

____

____

____

____

____

____

____

____

____

____

____

____

____

❖ Name three herbs mentioned in the chapter that are known for their ability to support liver function and aid in detoxification.

____

____

____

❖ Provide a step-by-step guide to preparing Milk Thistle Tea
and Turmeric Tea, and discuss how these teas can
contribute to improving liver function.

❖ Why is reducing exposure to common toxins through
lifestyle changes emphasized in combating symptoms
associated with Alzheimer's disease and Dementia, and
what are some examples of such lifestyle changes?

❖ Parkinson9s Disease

Parkinson's disease is a neurodegenerative disorder that primarily affects movement, characterized by symptoms such as tremors, stiffness, and difficulty with balance and coordination. The root cause of the disease lies in the loss of nerve cells in the substantia nigra of the brain, leading to a decrease in dopamine levels, a chemical crucial for controlling movement.

Herbal remedies, including Ginkgo biloba, Mucuna pruriens (containing L-DOPA, a dopamine precursor), and antioxidants, are suggested to manage these symptoms. The process of making a herbal potion involves steeping the specific herb in boiling water or infusing it into oil.

Reflection and exercises:

"   Who was James Parkinson, and what significant contribution did he make to the understanding of the disease now known as Parkinson's disease?

❖ Explain the root cause of Parkinson's disease, focusing on the role of nerve cells in the substantia nigra and the impact on dopamine levels.

❖ Name three herbal remedies mentioned in the chapter for managing Parkinson's disease symptoms and briefly describe their potential benefits.

____

____

____

____

____

____

____

____

____

❖ Provide a step-by-step guide to preparing a herbal tea with Mucuna pruriens, emphasizing the importance of this herb in the context of Parkinson's disease management.

____

____

____

____

____

____

____

____

____

____

❖ **Multiple Sclerosis and Amyotrophic Lateral Sclerosis**

Multiple Sclerosis (MS) and Amyotrophic Lateral Sclerosis (ALS) are attributed primarily to fluke parasites in the brain or spinal cord, worsened by solvents like xylene and toluene, Shigella bacteria from dairy products, and mercury from dental metals. Proposed solutions involve using a zapper or frequency generator to kill parasites, avoiding specific foods, sterilizing dairy products rigorously, and performing kidney and liver cleanses.

The root cause of these conditions is the invasion of fluke parasites facilitated by solvents, Shigella bacteria, and mercury pollution from dental metals. Natural remedies include anti-parasitic herbs like wormwood and black walnut hulls, detoxifying herbs like milk thistle and dandelion root, and nervous system-supporting herbs like ashwagandha and ginkgo biloba. Herbal potions include anti-parasitic tincture, liver detox tea, and nervous system support tea.

Reflections and exercises:

❖ Identify three contributing factors to the development of Multiple Sclerosis (MS) and Amyotrophic Lateral Sclerosis (ALS) as mentioned in the chapter.

❖ Explain the role of anti-parasitic herbs, detoxifying herbs, and nervous system-supporting herbs in the proposed natural remedies for MS and ALS.

❖ Provide a step-by-step guide to preparing the Anti-Parasitic Tincture mentioned in the chapter, and discuss its recommended usage

❖ How can avoiding specific foods, rigorous sterilization of dairy products, and kidney and liver cleanses contribute to managing MS and ALS symptoms based on the information provided in the chapter?

❖ Epilepsy

Epilepsy, historically known as the "falling sickness," was once believed to be linked to dietary missteps causing bowel obstruction and nerve disturbances. This could lead to altered blood flow to the brain and various physical symptoms. However, contemporary understanding recognizes epilepsy as possibly hereditary, emerging in childhood and persisting throughout life, or as a result of brain injuries, tumors, or infections. The root cause of epilepsy is considered to be either genetic predisposition or physical factors.

Herbal remedies for epilepsy focus on antispasmodic properties and overall nervous system support, with herbs like black cohosh, valerian, lady's slipper, and skullcap recommended for their calming and nerve-supportive qualities. An herbal tea can be prepared by steeping a blend of these herbs in boiling water and drinking it when an impending attack is sensed. Additional recommendations include maintaining a nourishing diet, avoiding stimulants and constipating foods, and ensuring bowel health through enemas to complement the herbal treatment.

Reflections and exercises:

❖ Explain the historical beliefs regarding the causes of epilepsy, including dietary missteps and nerve disturbances, and contrast them with contemporary understanding.

____

____

____

____

____

____

____

____

____

____

____

____

❖ Name four herbs mentioned in the chapter for their antispasmodic properties and nerve-supportive qualities in managing epilepsy.

____

____

❖ Provide a step-by-step guide to preparing the herbal tea mentioned in the chapter for epilepsy, and discuss when it is recommended to be consumed.

❖ Stroke

Stroke, a leading cause of paralysis and death, results from reduced blood flow to the brain due to arterial blockages or ruptured vessels. Symptoms may include complete or partial body paralysis, speech impairment, and unresponsiveness to physical stimuli. Immediate and effective treatment is crucial, with traditional methods like hot and cold fomentations, massage, liniments, and specific herbs showing success.

The root cause of strokes leading to paralysis is the disruption of normal blood circulation to the brain, often caused by plaque formation in the arteries or the rupture of a blood vessel within the brain. Natural remedies for stroke recovery include herbs such as Masterwort, Black Cohosh, Hyssop, Vervain, Blue Cohosh, Catnip, an antispasmodic tincture, and Skullcap, known for their properties that may aid in circulation, reduce inflammation, and support nerve function. Herbal potions can be prepared using a combination of these herbs in a dried or fresh form, steeped in boiling water to create a tea for consumption 2-3 times a day.

Reflections and exercises:

❖ Describe the symptoms of a stroke mentioned in the chapter, emphasizing the impact on an individual's ability to move and speak.

❖ What are the primary causes of strokes leading to paralysis, and how do arterial blockages or ruptured vessels contribute to this condition?

____

____

❖ Provide a step-by-step guide to preparing the herbal potion
for stroke recovery mentioned in the chapter, including the
selection and preparation of herbs and the recommended
usage.

____

____

____

____

____

____

____

____

____

____

____

____

____

____

____

❖ Myasthenia Gravis

Myasthenia Gravis is a condition characterized by muscle weakness, particularly in the eyelids, and is believed to be influenced by a chemical possibly originating from a parasitic fluke. This chemical may trigger an allergic reaction, affecting acetylcholine receptors and leading to muscle inefficiency. The thymus gland, highly sensitive to benzene, a prevalent toxin, is often implicated. Addressing this condition involves a comprehensive approach, including eliminating parasites and bacteria, reducing exposure to toxins, and maintaining a strict herbal parasite program.

The root cause of Myasthenia Gravis appears to be a combination of parasitic infection (flukes) and exposure to toxins like benzene, disrupting the normal functioning of acetylcholine receptors crucial for muscle control. Herbal remedies focus on eradicating parasites and detoxifying the body, with herbs like wormwood, black walnut hulls, cloves, milk thistle, and dandelion root recommended. Herbal potions include antiparasitic and detoxifying blends, consumed regularly as part of the treatment plan

Reflection and exercises:

❖ Explain the possible root causes of Myasthenia Gravis, including the role of parasitic infection and exposure to toxins like benzene.

____

____

____

____

____

____

❖ Name three herbs mentioned in the chapter known for their anti-parasitic properties and their potential effectiveness in addressing Myasthenia Gravis.

❖ Provide a step-by-step guide to preparing the anti-parasitic potion and detoxifying potion mentioned in the chapter, and discuss their recommended usage.

____

____

____

____

____

____

____

❖ Why is it emphasized in the chapter that both the affected individual and their family should adopt measures to ensure a parasite-free environment for managing Myasthenia Gravis?

____

____

____

____

____

____

____

____

❖ Hydrocephalus

Hydrocephalus, commonly known as "water on the brain," is characterized by an abnormal accumulation of cerebrospinal fluid (CSF) within the brain's ventricles, leading to increased pressure inside the skull. This condition can be congenital, present at birth due to genetic factors or developmental disorders like spina bifida, or acquired later in life due to infections, injuries, or brain tumors.

Herbal remedies for hydrocephalus traditionally include various herbs like sage, rue, rosemary, calamus, broom, catnip, red sage, marjoram, woodbetony, pennyroyal, skullcap, and calamint. To prepare a herbal potion, one can select and clean the herbs, boil water, steep the herbs in hot water, simmer for 10-15 minutes, strain the mixture, and allow it to cool before storage in the refrigerator.

Reflections and exercises:

❖ Explain the root causes of hydrocephalus and how they can vary from congenital factors to acquired conditions later in life.

____

____

____

____

____

____

____

____

____

____

____

____

____

❖ Name at least five herbs traditionally used in herbal preparations for hydrocephalus, and briefly discuss their potential benefits.

❖ Provide a step-by-step guide to preparing a herbal potion for hydrocephalus using the mentioned herbs, emphasizing the proper ratios and simmering time.

❖ Discuss the potential challenges and considerations in using herbal remedies for hydrocephalus, especially in cases where the cause is unknown.

PART V: GASTRO INTESTINAL & DIGESTIVE DISORDERS

The upcoming series of chapters delves into the effectiveness of herbal remedies in addressing a spectrum of gastrointestinal and digestive disorders. From common issues like indigestion and gastritis to more complex conditions such as irritable bowel syndrome (IBS) and inflammatory bowel disease (IBD), these chapters explore the roots of these disorders and offer insights into natural remedies drawn from traditional herbal knowledge. As we navigate through each chapter, we'll uncover the potential benefits of herbs in promoting digestive health and alleviating associated symptoms.

❖ Gastro-esophageal Reflux Disease (GERD)

Gastro-esophageal Reflux Disease (GERD), commonly known as acid reflux, is a chronic condition characterized by the regurgitation of stomach contents into the esophagus, leading to symptoms or complications. While modern medicine labels it as GERD, historical references have recognized similar symptoms under different names such as heartburn or acid indigestion. The root cause of GERD lies in the malfunction of the lower esophageal sphincter (LES), allowing stomach acid to flow back into the esophagus due to weakness or inappropriate relaxation of the sphincter. Lifestyle choices, dietary habits, obesity, and certain medications contribute to this dysfunction.

Natural remedies, rooted in centuries-old herbal traditions, offer a holistic approach to managing GERD. Various herbs, including Beech, Calamus, Golden Seal, Ginger, and many more, have been historically praised for their medicinal properties. Creating a herbal potion involves steeping these herbs in hot water to extract their beneficial compounds, providing potential relief from GERD symptoms.

Reflections and exercises

❖ How does GERD differ from historical descriptions of
similar conditions like heartburn or acid indigestion?

____

____

____

____

____

____

____

____

____

____

____

____

❖ Explain the role of the lower esophageal sphincter (LES) in
GERD, and how its malfunction contributes to the
condition.

____

____

____

____

____

____

____

____

____

____

____

____

____

____

____

____

❖ Discuss the significance of lifestyle choices in the
development of GERD and how they impact the lower
esophageal sphincter.

____

____

____

____

____

____

____

____

____

____

❖ Choose three herbs from the provided list and elaborate on
their traditional medicinal properties believed to be
beneficial for GERD.

____

____

____

____

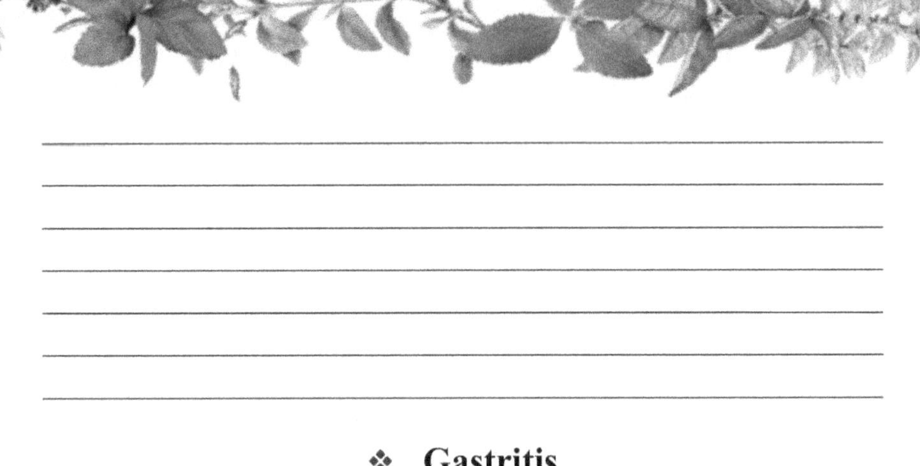

____

____

____

____

____

____

____

❖ Gastritis

Gastritis, marked by inflammation in the stomach lining, stems from lifestyle decisions and various medical conditions. Triggers encompass alcohol use, consistent intake of anti-inflammatory medications like aspirin, and exposure to strong acids or alkalis, sometimes linked to suicide attempts or accidental ingestion by children. The condition is further aggravated by the consumption of spicy foods and condiments, leading to symptoms such as upper abdominal pain, nausea, vomiting, appetite loss, weight loss, gas, and a burning sensation. Contemporary management involves steering clear of irritants, embracing a mild and nutritious diet, and integrating soothing herbal remedies.

The central causes of gastritis involve alcohol, specific medications (especially aspirin), and the consumption of overly spicy or stimulating foods, all of which induce inflammation in the stomach lining, causing discomfort and varied symptoms. Herbal solutions like goldenseal, sage, wood betony, slippery elm, along with red raspberry tea and chickweed tea, have demonstrated efficacy in providing natural relief. A herbal concoction consisting of golden seal, echinacea, burnet, wood betony, myrrh, and spearmint, when taken before meals and bedtime, offers substantial relief from the symptoms associated with gastritis.

Reflections and exercises:

❖ Elaborate on how lifestyle choices and medical conditions contribute to the onset of gastritis.

____

____

____

____

____

____

____

____

____

____

____

____

❖ Analyze the impact of common triggers like alcohol, aspirin, and spicy foods in instigating inflammation in the stomach lining.

____

____

____

____

____

____

____

____

____

____

❖ Describe the symptoms linked with gastritis and their implications for an individual's overall health.

❖ Assess the effectiveness of herbal remedies in addressing gastritis and the pharmaceutical industry's stance on herbal treatments.

❖ Crohn9s Disease

Crohn's Disease, a form of inflammatory bowel disease (IBD) affecting any part of the gastrointestinal tract, was first described by Dr. Burrill B. Crohn in 1932. Often confused with ulcerative colitis, another IBD variant confined to the colon and rectum, its exact cause remains elusive. Factors such as genetics, immune system aberrations, and environmental triggers are believed to contribute, with stress and diet exacerbating but not causing the condition.

While herbal remedies have historical use and believers in their efficacy, their application in treating Crohn's Disease lacks widespread scientific backing. Traditionally used herbs include Aloe Vera, Turmeric (Curcumin), Slippery Elm, and Peppermint Oil. The herbal potion-making process involves herb selection based on symptoms, preparation through steeping or mixing, and cautious dosage. Consultation with healthcare providers is essential due to the complexity of Crohn's Disease, and while some assert the underestimation of herbal potential by pharmaceutical companies, a critical and informed approach is advised.

Reflections and exercises:

❖ Have you ever suffered Crohn9s disease? If yes, describe, in detail, how you felt and managed it.

____

____

____

____

____

____

❖ Outline the factors believed to contribute to the development of Crohn's Disease and its complex nature.

❖ Evaluate the historical use of herbal remedies in managing symptoms akin to Crohn's Disease and the current scientific support for their efficacy.

____

____

____

____

____

____

____

____

____

____

____

❖ Irritable Bowel Syndrome (IBS)

Irritable Bowel Syndrome (IBS), Colitis, and Spastic Colon, viewed as complex conditions, are now associated with a blend of parasitic, bacterial issues, and potential allergic reactions. While traditional understanding attributed these conditions to specific food triggers, the modern perspective emphasizes underlying infections like Salmonella or Shigella, toxins, and pancreas parasites as potential causes.

The holistic approach to cure involves eliminating parasites, bacteria, and viruses, coupled with lifestyle modifications such as dietary changes and environmental clean-up.

Reflection and exercises:

❖ Reflect on your personal experiences with herbs in managing digestive issues. How have herbs like Black Walnut Hull Tincture Extra Strength or others contributed to alleviating symptoms or promoting well-being?

____
____
____
____
____
____
____
____
____
____

❖ Share instances where dietary modifications and environmental changes, coupled with herbal remedies, have positively impacted your digestive health. What herbs, in particular, have you found effective in your own journey?

____
____
____
____
____
____
____
____

❖   Discuss the challenges you've encountered in incorporating herbal potions or remedies into your lifestyle for conditions like Irritable Bowel Syndrome (IBS), Colitis, or Spastic Colon. What strategies have proven helpful in overcoming these challenges?

❖ Appendicitis

Appendicitis is often linked to poor dietary choices, particularly the excessive consumption of processed foods and stimulants. The condition results from a blockage in the appendix, leading to inflammation and potential infections. Immediate relief can be sought through herbal enemas for colon cleansing, while long-term management involves a liquid diet with alkaline broths and herbal teas. However, in acute cases, seeking immediate medical attention is crucial.

Reflections and exercises:

❖ Share instances from your own experience or someone you know where herbal remedies were utilized for digestive issues. How effective were these remedies, and what herbs were involved?

____

____

____

____

____

____

____

____

____

____

____

____

❖ Reflect on your dietary habits. Have you observed a connection between your food choices, especially processed foods and stimulants, and your digestive health? How might modifying these habits positively impact your well-being?

____

____

____

____

❖ If you have tried herbal potions for digestive concerns, what herbs did you find most beneficial, and how did you incorporate them into your routine? Share any challenges or successes.

❖ Considering the recommendation for immediate medical attention in acute cases of appendicitis, how do you navigate the balance between herbal remedies and conventional medical care in managing digestive disorders? What factors influence your decision-making in this regard?

❖ Hernia

Hiatal hernia, a condition where part of the stomach protrudes through the diaphragm, commonly affects individuals over 50. While the exact cause is unclear, factors like age, obesity, and smoking contribute. Behaviors such as overeating and lying down after meals can exacerbate it. Natural remedies involve herbs like slippery elm, marshmallow root, and chamomile, known for their soothing properties on the digestive system.

Reflections and exercises:

❖ Considering risk factors like age and obesity, what preventive measures can be incorporated into one's lifestyle to potentially reduce the risk of developing a hiatal hernia?

____

____

____

____

____

____

____

____

____

____

____

____

____

____

❖ How do specific behaviors like overeating or lying down after meals affect digestive health, and how might modifying these behaviors contribute to managing or preventing hiatal hernias?

____

____

____

____

❖ Share any personal experiences or stories you know about using herbal remedies, such as slippery elm or chamomile, for digestive issues. What were the outcomes?

❖ Gall stones

Gallstones, prevalent among middle-aged, overweight individuals, are influenced by factors such as a high-calorie, high-fat diet, and specific lifestyle choices. While their exact cause remains elusive, dietary habits play a significant role. Herbs like Bitterroot, Cascara Sagrada, and Chamomile have been effective in treating gallstones, offering a natural alternative to pharmaceutical solutions. Herbal potions, including tea mixtures and olive oil-citrus juice blends, aim to support gallstone elimination. These remedies, rooted in nature, echo the philosophy of seeking cures from natural sources.

Reflections and exercises:

❖ How might adopting a low-fat diet and avoiding specific foods contribute to preventing or managing gallstones, based on the information provided?

____

____

____

____

____

____

____

____

____

____

❖ In your opinion, how do herbal remedies like Bitterroot and Cascara Sagrada compare to pharmaceutical solutions for gallstones? Consider factors like effectiveness, side effects, and overall impact.

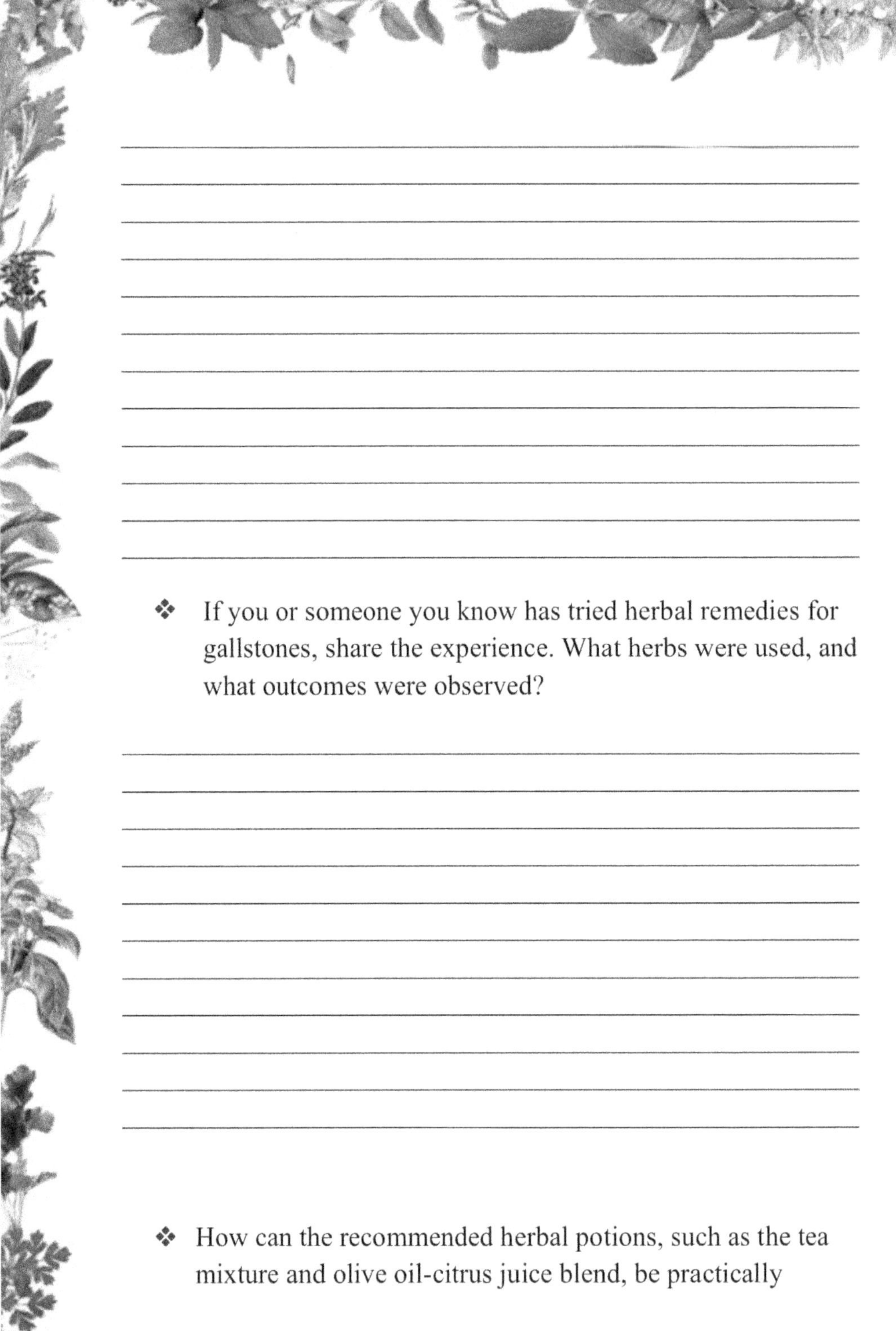

❖ If you or someone you know has tried herbal remedies for gallstones, share the experience. What herbs were used, and what outcomes were observed?

❖ How can the recommended herbal potions, such as the tea mixture and olive oil-citrus juice blend, be practically integrated into a daily routine? Are there any challenges or considerations in following these remedies consistently?

____

____

____

____

____

____

____

____

____

____

❖ Hepatitis

Hepatitis, characterized by liver inflammation, can result from various factors, with viruses, toxins, medications, and autoimmune diseases being common causes. Chronic hepatitis, particularly types B and C, may lead to severe conditions like liver cirrhosis and cancer. Some believe in the potential of herbal remedies, including milk thistle, licorice root, and dandelion, for liver protection. However, it's essential to note that these remedies lack universal acceptance in the medical community. Creating herbal potions, such as teas from milk thistle or dandelion, is a method attempted by those seeking natural alternatives for hepatitis.

Reflections and exercises:

❖   Reflect on your understanding of viral hepatitis. If you were to explain it to a friend, how would you describe the impact of hepatitis A, B, C, D, and E on liver inflammation? What questions might your friend ask?

____
____
____
____
____
____
____
____
____
____

❖   Have you ever been curious about herbal remedies like milk thistle, licorice root, or dandelion for liver health? What information or experiences led you to consider or question their effectiveness?

____
____
____
____
____
____

❖ Share any personal encounters or stories you've come across regarding individuals trying herbal remedies for hepatitis. How did these experiences shape your perception of natural treatments?

❖ If you've considered or used herbal treatments, what factors influenced your decision? Did you consult with a healthcare provider, and how did the integration of herbal remedies impact your overall health journey?

____

____

____

____

____

____

____

____

❖ Smoking Addiction

Tobacco use, whether through smoking or chewing, poses significant health risks, including various cancers and heart-related issues. The root cause lies in the harmful toxins present in tobacco, adversely affecting the entire body. A natural remedy involves a detoxifying diet, hot baths, and herbal teas like red clover, magnolia, myrtle, slippery elm, and others, aiming not only for detoxification but also for overall health improvement.

Reflections and exercises:

- ❖ If you were to embark on a detox journey to overcome smoking addiction, what challenges do you anticipate, and how might herbal teas like red clover or magnolia play a role in supporting your journey?

____

____

____

____

____

____

____

❖ Jaundice

Jaundice is marked by yellowing of the skin and eyes, and results from an obstruction in the liver or bile ducts, causing excess bile absorption into the blood. Root causes include liver diseases, gallstones, infections, or certain medications. Traditional treatments involve fruit juices like lemon and grapefruit for detoxification and herbal teas using dandelion, milk thistle, turmeric, barberry, chicory, and yellow dock for relief.

Reflections and exercises:

❖ How comfortable are you incorporating herbs like dandelion, milk thistle, or turmeric into your daily routine to promote liver health, considering their potential benefits for conditions like jaundice?

❖ Before reading this, how much did you know about jaundice and its natural remedies? How has this information influenced your understanding of alternative approaches to liver-related conditions?

____

____

____

____

____

____

____

____

❖ If you were to create your herbal potion for jaundice, which herbs would you choose based on your preferences or accessibility? How do you think personalizing herbal remedies can enhance their effectiveness?

____

____

____

____

____

____

____

____

____

____

❖ In managing jaundice, how comfortable are you combining
traditional approaches, like herbal potions, with modern
medical advice? What factors would influence your
decision to integrate both?

____

____

____

____

____

❖ All Liver Cancers

Liver disease, encompassing conditions like hepatitis, cirrhosis,
liver cancer, and fatty liver disease, arises from various factors
such as viral infections, alcohol abuse, fatty liver, autoimmune
disorders, genetic issues, and exposure to toxins. Herbal remedies,
including a wide range of herbs like bitterroot, milk thistle,
dandelion, and more, have been traditionally used for liver health.
However, caution is advised due to varying scientific evidence.
The chapter emphasizes considering both traditional knowledge
and scientific evidence when exploring herbal treatments for liver
issues.

Reflections and exercises

❖ Before reading this chapter, how familiar were you with the
potential herbal remedies for liver diseases? Has your
understanding of herbal treatments for liver health evolved?

____

____

____

____

____

____

❖ Considering the diverse causes of liver diseases, how comfortable are you blending traditional herbal remedies with modern medical advice in managing liver health? What factors would influence your approach?

❖ If you were to create a herbal potion for liver health, which herbs would you choose based on your understanding and potential benefits? How might personalizing herbal remedies enhance their effectiveness for you?

❖ The chapter discusses the notion that pharmaceutical companies may downplay herbal remedies. How do you balance the use of herbal remedies with pharmaceuticals, considering both have their merits?

❖ **Tumor**

Reflections and Exercises:

" Have you ever wondered how tumors form in the body, and what impact they might have on your health?

❖ Share any personal experiences or stories you've heard about tumor treatment. What approaches were effective?

❖ If you had to explain tumors to a friend, how would you describe them in simple terms?

❖ **Inflamed Pancreas**

Reflections and Exercises:

❖ Ever felt curious about the pancreas and its role in digestion? Let's dive into why it matters!

❖ If you've heard of inflammation affecting the pancreas, what lifestyle habits do you think could contribute to this issue?

____

____

____

____

____

____

____

____

❖   Imagine you're exploring holistic health 3 what dietary changes would you consider to support your pancreas?

____

____

____

____

____

____

____

____

____

❖   **Colitis**

Reflections and Exercises:

❖ Personal stories can be powerful. Do you know anyone who has dealt with colitis, and how did they manage it?

____

____

____

____

____

____

____

____

❖ Picture yourself in control of your colitis management plan. What dietary changes would you be excited to try?

____

____

____

____

____

____

____

____

❖ Herbal remedies often have unique benefits. If you were to explore natural options for colitis, where would you start?

____

____

____

____

____

____

____

____

____

____

❖ Stomach Cancer

Reflections and Exercises:

❖ Health journeys are unique. Have you or someone you
know faced risks associated with stomach cancer?

____

____

____

____

____

____

____

____

____

____

❖ Imagine you're part of a support group. What insights
would you share about stomach cancer symptoms and
early detection?

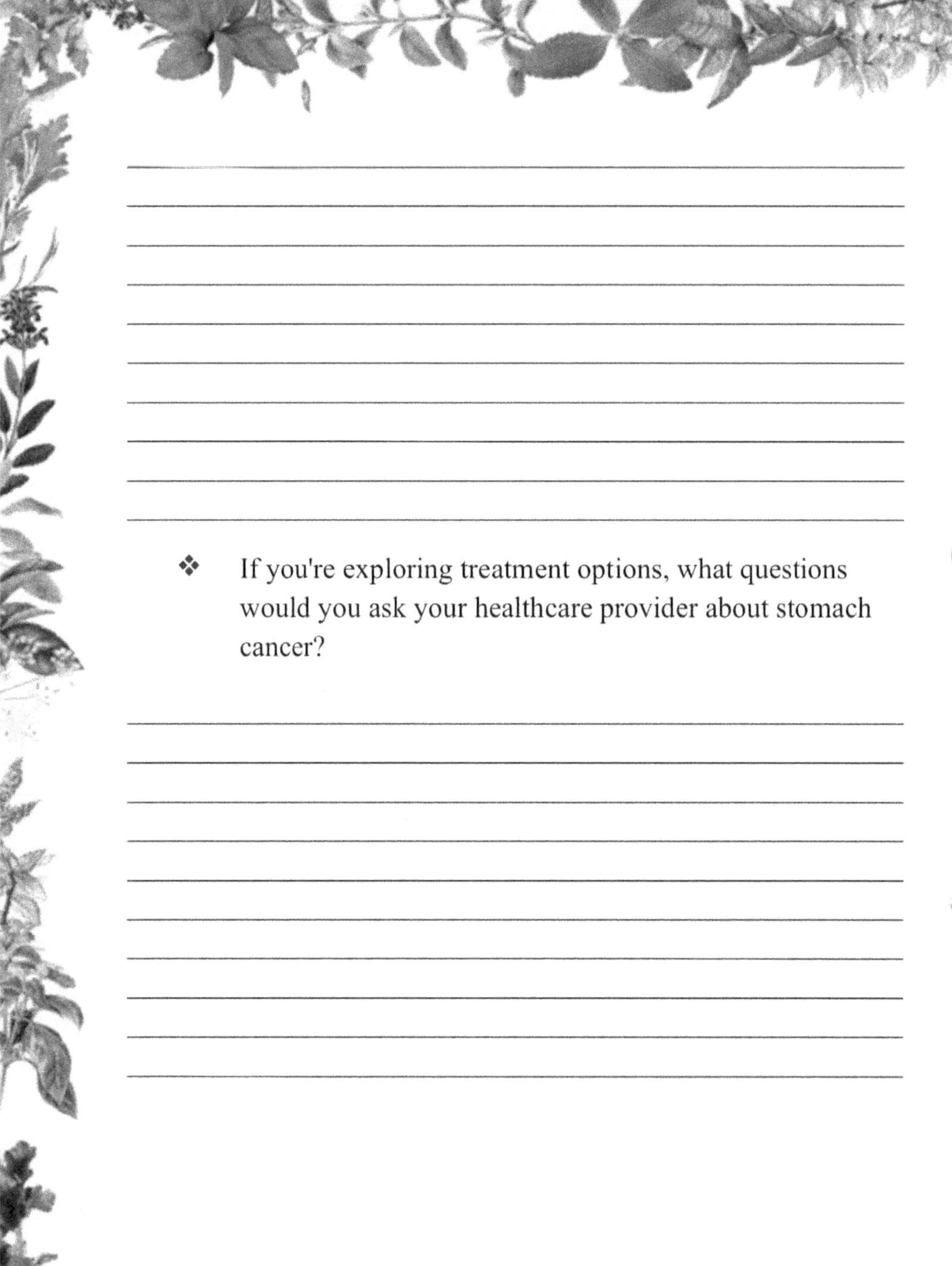

❖ If you're exploring treatment options, what questions would you ask your healthcare provider about stomach cancer?

❖ **Piles**

Reflections and Exercises:

❖ Let's make it relatable 3 have you ever experienced the discomfort of piles, or know someone who has?

____

____

____

____

____

____

____

____

❖ Healthy habits matter! What lifestyle changes would you consider to prevent and manage piles?

____

____

____

____

____

____

____

____

____

❖ Herbal remedies can be intriguing. If you were to try a natural approach for piles, which herbs would you be curious about?

____

____

____

____

____

____

____

____

____

❖ Anal Fissures

Reflections and Exercises:

❖ Anal fissures might be more common than we think. Any personal tips or experiences you'd share to manage them?

____

____

____

____

____

❖ Lifestyle changes can make a big difference. What habits would you adopt to prevent and care for anal fissures?

❖ If you're into holistic health, which herbal remedies might you explore for anal fissures?

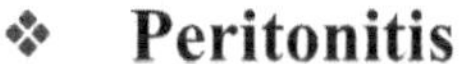 **Peritonitis**

Reflections and Exercises:

❖ Health scares happen. Have you ever wondered about peritonitis and how it occurs?

____

____

____

____

____

____

____

____

❖ Thinking prevention, what daily habits would you adopt to steer clear of peritonitis risks?

____

____

____

____

____

____

____

❖ Picture yourself as a health advocate. What advice would you give your friends about avoiding peritonitis?

____

____

____

____

____

____

____

____

____

____

Croup

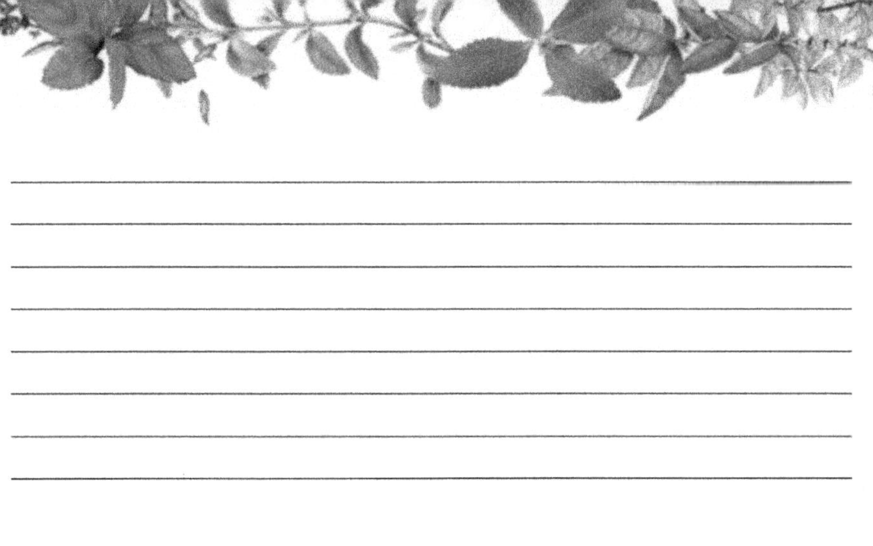

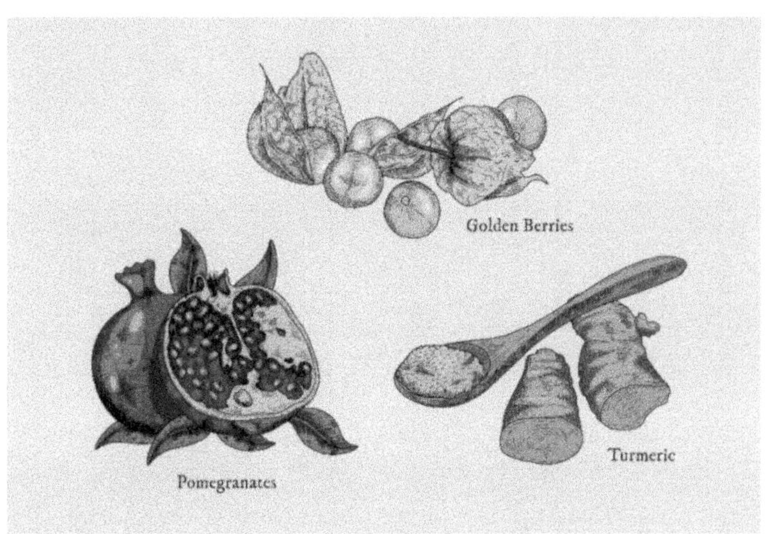

Reflections and exercises:

❖ Parents, ever faced croup with your little ones? Share your experiences and tips!

____

____

____

❖ Home remedies can be comforting. What tried-and-true methods have you used or heard about for managing croup?

❖ If you were part of a parenting forum, what advice would you offer to others dealing with croup?

Stomach Gas

Reflections and exercises:

❖ Let's talk real life! Stomach gas can be common. Any funny or interesting anecdotes about dealing with it?

____
____
____
____
____
____
____
____
____

❖ Health is personal. What lifestyle changes would you consider to reduce stomach gas and improve digestion?

____
____
____
____
____
____
____

Herbal remedies are intriguing. If you were to experiment with natural solutions, which herbs might you try?

Blood Poisoning

Reflections and Exercises:

- ❖ Scary but essential 3 have you ever come across stories or information about blood poisoning?

❖ Quick responses matter. What immediate steps would you take if you suspected blood poisoning?

❖ In a wellness community, what preventative measures and herbal tips would you share to keep the blood healthy?

PART VI: RESPIRATORY DISEASES

Asthma

Reflections and Exercises:

❖ Asthma can be a challenging companion. Have you or someone close to you experienced the struggles of asthma? Share personal stories or insights that have shaped your understanding of living with this respiratory condition.

____

____

____

____

____

____

____

____

____

____

❖ Imagine a sudden asthma attack. What immediate relief strategies, including herbal remedies or calming practices, would you employ to ease breathing difficulties? Share how you would apply the steps stipulated in the book.

____

____

____

____

____

____

____

____

Cough and cold

Reflections and exercises:

"	Coughs and colds are universal experiences. What are your personal coping mechanisms when faced with a persistent cough or cold? Share your favorite herbal remedies, comfort foods, or activities that help you navigate through these common respiratory challenges.

____
____
____
____
____
____
____
____

❖ How would you creatively use herbs to prepare immune-boosting recipes to combat coughs and colds?

____
____
____
____
____
____

❖ Picture yourself curating winter wellness herbal kits for your friends and family. What herbal preparations, like teas or soothing balms, would you include to support respiratory health during the colder months? Share your personalized approach to gifting wellness in a kit.

____
____
____

____

____

____

____

____

____

____

Pneumonia

Reflections and exercises:

❖ Pneumonia can be a serious health setback. Have you or
someone you know faced the challenges of pneumonia?
Share your personal encounters or stories related to
pneumonia and how it influenced your perspective on
respiratory health.

____

____

____

____

____

____

____

____

____

❖ Envision a personalized recovery plan for overcoming
pneumonia. What specific herbal remedies or wellness
rituals would you incorporate to support a swift and

effective recovery? Share insights into crafting a holistic approach to pneumonia healing.

____

____

____

____

____

____

____

____

- ❖ If you were leading a virtual support group for individuals recovering from pneumonia, how would you foster a sense of community and share practical herbal tips for a smooth recovery journey? Consider the unique experiences and insights you'd bring to the virtual gathering

____

____

____

____

____

____

____

____

____

Pleurisy

Reflections and exercises:

❖ Pleurisy can bring sharp chest pains. Have you encountered pleurisy personally or through someone you know? Share any insights, experiences, or knowledge you've gained about dealing with pleurisy and its impact on respiratory health

____

____

____

____

____

____

____

____

____

❖ In the face of pleuritic pain, what herbal or natural measures would you recommend to bring comfort and relief as recommended in the book?

____

____

____

____

____

____

____

____

____

Chronic Bronchitis

Reflections and exercises:

❖ Chronic bronchitis can be persistent. Have you or someone close to you navigated the challenges of chronic bronchitis? Share personal experiences or stories that have shaped your understanding of living with this chronic respiratory condition.

____

____

____

____

____

____

____

____

____

❖ What herbs and lifestyle practices would you incorporate to support consistent respiratory well-being?

____

____

____

____

____

____

____

____

Catarrh

Reflections and exercises:

❖ How do you understand catarrh?

____

____

____

____

____

❖ What experiences or knowledge do you have about dealing
with excess mucus in the respiratory system?

____

____

____

____

____

❖ Share insights or personal stories that have contributed to
your awareness of catarrh.

____

____

____

____

____

❖ In times of increased catarrh, what herbal solutions or natural remedies would you turn to for relief? Share your favorite herbs or preparations that effectively address catarrh symptoms and promote respiratory comfort.

____

____

____

____

____

____

____

____

____

Coli (in infants)

Reflections and exercises:

❖ Coli in infants can be concerning for parents. Have you or someone close to you dealt with coli in infants?

____

____

____

____

____

____

____

❖ Share parenting insights, experiences, or supportive
   measures you've learned to address coli and ensure the
   well-being of infants.

____

____

____

____

____

____

❖ Imagine creating a herbal comfort kit for infants
   experiencing coli. What herbal remedies or soothing
   measures would you include to provide relief for both
   infants and their parents?

____

____

____

____

____

____

Influenza

Reflections and exercises:

❖ Share a personal experience or encounter with influenza.
   How did it impact your daily life, and what measures did
   you take to manage the symptoms?

____

____

____

____

____

❖ Explore the diverse herbal remedies mentioned for
   influenza. Which herbs resonate with you, and have you
   tried any of them before? Share your insights or
   experiences with herbal treatments for respiratory illnesses.

____

____

____

____

____

❖ Discuss preventive measures against influenza mentioned
   in the chapter. What steps do you take to prevent the flu in

your daily life, especially during peak flu seasons or in challenging environmental conditions?

____

____

____

____

____

❖ The chapter emphasizes the importance of bed rest, fluid intake, and fresh air for continued care during influenza. How do you take care of yourself or others when symptoms persist? Share practical strategies for providing comfort and support.

____

____

____

____

____

PART VII: ENDOCRINE AND METABOLLIC DISORDERS

Ricket

Reflections and exercises:

❖ How familiar are you with the condition of rickets? Share any prior knowledge or experiences you have regarding this disease.

____
____
____
____
____
____

❖ Explore the nutritional aspects discussed for managing rickets. What dietary changes or supplements would you recommend to someone looking to prevent or address rickets? Share your insights into the role of nutrition in bone health.

____
____
____
____
____
____

❖ Sun exposure is crucial for vitamin D synthesis, a key factor in preventing rickets. How do you incorporate sun exposure into your routine, and what advice would you give to others regarding safe sun practices?

Goiter

Reflections and exercises:

- ❖ How would you explain goiter to someone unfamiliar with the condition? Share any experiences or knowledge you have regarding the causes and symptoms of goiter.

- ❖ Delve into the herbal remedies mentioned for goiter, such as bladderwrack and dulse. Have you tried any of these herbs, and how do you incorporate them into your routine? Share your insights into herbal support for thyroid health.

- ❖ Explore the importance of iodine in preventing and managing goiter. What iodine-rich foods would you include in your diet, and how do you ensure an adequate intake of this essential mineral?

____

____

____

____

____

❖ If you were leading a community awareness campaign on goiter prevention, what creative initiatives and communication strategies would you use to inform people about the role of iodine and herbs in maintaining a healthy thyroid?

____

____

____

____

____

____

Gout

Reflections and exercises:

❖ Share any personal experiences or encounters with gout, either firsthand or through someone you know. How did it impact daily life, and what measures were taken to manage the symptoms?

❖ Explore the dietary recommendations for managing gout.
What dietary changes would you adopt or suggest to
someone looking to alleviate gout symptoms? Share your
insights into the role of nutrition in gout management.

❖ Delve into the herbal remedies mentioned for gout, such as
yarrow, skull cap, valerian, ginger, blue violet, broom,
birch, balm of Gilead etc. Have you tried any of these
herbs, and how do you integrate them into your approach to
managing gout? Share your experiences with herbal
support for joint health.

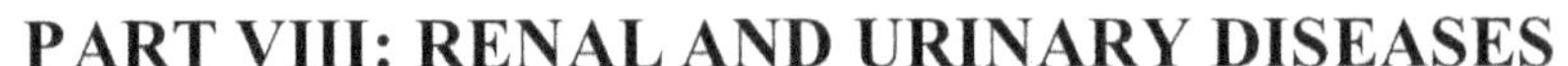

PART VIII: RENAL AND URINARY DISEASES

Dropsy or Edema

Reflections and exercises:

- ❖ How would you explain dropsy or edema to someone unfamiliar with the condition? Share any experiences or knowledge you have regarding the causes and symptoms of dropsy.

____

____

____

____

____

____

____

____

❖ Explore the dietary recommendations for managing dropsy. What dietary changes would you adopt or suggest to someone dealing with edema? Share your insights into the role of nutrition in fluid balance.

____

____

____

____

____

____

❖ Delve into the herbal remedies mentioned for dropsy such as red raspberry and pleurisy root teas a. Have you tried any of these herbs, and how do you incorporate them into your routine? Share your experiences with herbal support for reducing fluid retention.

____

____

____

____

____

❖ Lifestyle plays a role in managing dropsy. What lifestyle adjustments would you recommend to someone dealing with edema? Discuss the importance of physical activity, sleep, and stress management in fluid balance.

____
____
____
____
____
____

Kidney Stones

Reflections and exercises:

❖ Share any personal experiences or encounters with kidney stones, either firsthand or through someone you know. How did it impact daily life, and what measures were taken to manage or prevent kidney stones?

____
____
____
____
____
____

❖ Explore the dietary recommendations for managing kidney stones. What dietary changes would you adopt or suggest to someone prone to kidney stones? Share your insights into the role of nutrition in kidney stone prevention.

❖ Delve into the herbal remedies mentioned for kidney stones, such as queen of the meadow, peach leaves, cleavers etc. Have you tried any of these herbs, and how do you integrate them into your approach to managing kidney stones? Share your experiences with herbal support for kidney health.

Bright 9s disease or Nephritis

❖ How would you explain Bright's disease or nephritis to someone unfamiliar with the condition? Share any

experiences or knowledge you have regarding the causes
and symptoms of Bright's disease.

____

____

____

____

____

❖ Explore the dietary recommendations for managing
Bright's disease. What dietary changes would you adopt or
suggest to someone dealing with nephritis? Share your
insights into the role of nutrition in kidney health.

____

____

____

____

____

____

Bladder Inflammation

❖ How would you explain cystitis or bladder inflammation to
someone unfamiliar with the condition? Share any
experiences or knowledge you have regarding the causes
and symptoms of cystitis.

____

____

____

- ❖ Explore the importance of hygiene in preventing cystitis.
  What hygiene practices do you prioritize, and how do they
  contribute to bladder health? Share your insights into
  maintaining cleanliness.

- ❖ Delve into the herbal remedies mentioned for cystitis, such
  as goldenrod and corn silk. Have you tried any of these
  herbs, and how do you integrate them into your routine?
  Share your experiences with herbal support for bladder
  inflammation.

❖ Adequate hydration is crucial for managing cystitis. How do you ensure proper hydration, and what advice would you offer to others regarding maintaining optimal fluid levels for bladder health?

PART IX: INFECTIOUS DISEASES

Diphtheria

❖ How familiar are you with diphtheria? Share any prior knowledge or experiences you have regarding this bacterial infection.

____

____

____

____

____

____

____

____

____

____

____

____

____

____

____

____

____

____

____

____

____

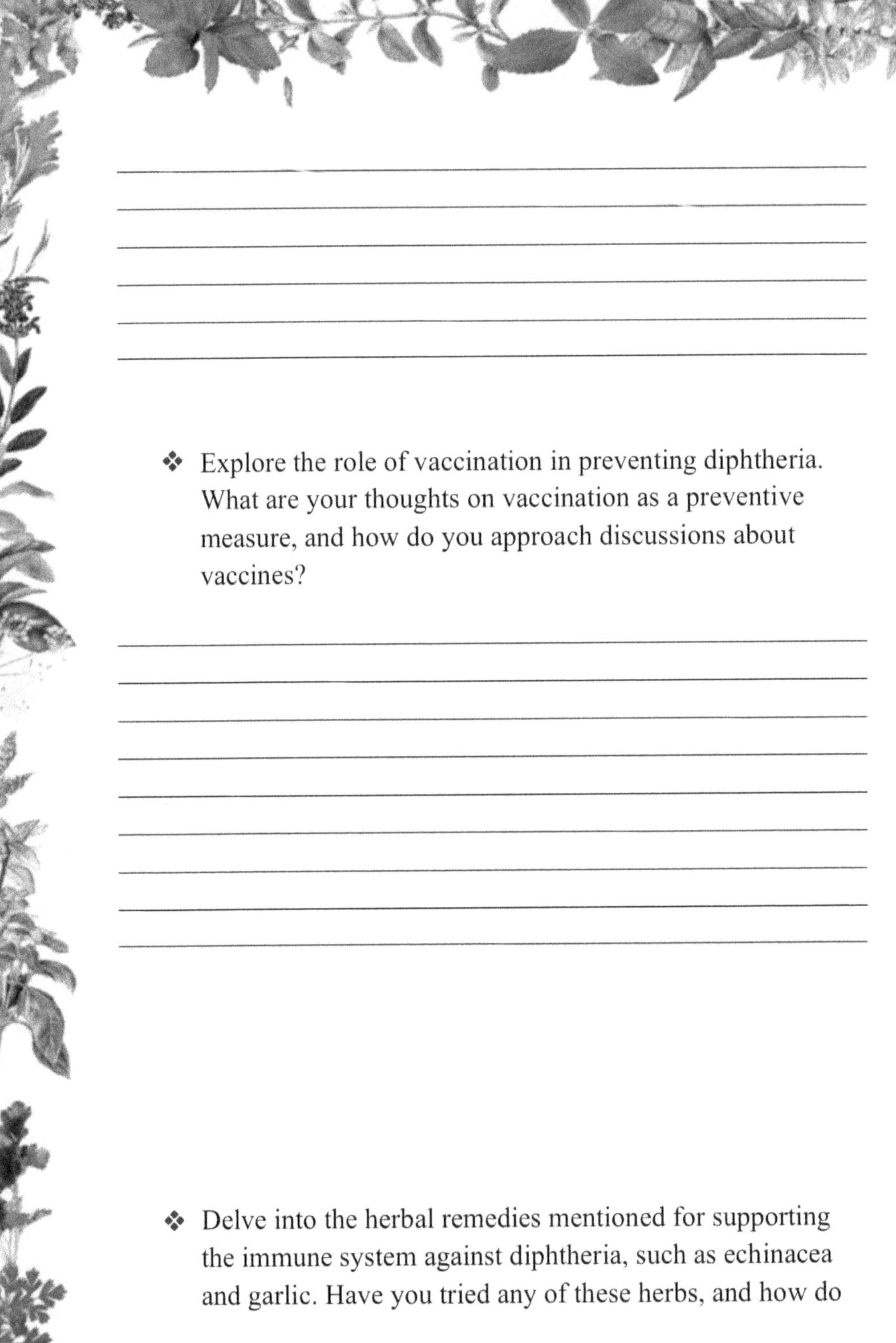

❖ Explore the role of vaccination in preventing diphtheria. What are your thoughts on vaccination as a preventive measure, and how do you approach discussions about vaccines?

❖ Delve into the herbal remedies mentioned for supporting the immune system against diphtheria, such as echinacea and garlic. Have you tried any of these herbs, and how do

you integrate them into your routine? Share your
experiences with herbal support for immune health.

____

____

____

____

____

____

____

____

____

In a community setting, what health practices would you promote
to prevent the spread of diphtheria? Discuss the importance of
community-wide efforts in controlling infectious diseases.

____

____

____

____

____

____

____

____

____

Tonsillitis

❖ Share any personal experiences or encounters with tonsillitis, either firsthand or through someone you know. How did it impact daily life, and what measures were taken to manage or prevent tonsillitis?

____

____

____

____

____

____

____

____

❖ Explore the home remedies mentioned for tonsillitis, such as warm saltwater gargles and chamomile. Have you tried any of these remedies, and how effective were they in relieving symptoms? Share your experiences with at-home tonsillitis management.

____

____

____

____

____

____

____

____

____

____

❖ How do you prioritize oral hygiene in preventing
tonsillitis? Discuss the importance of maintaining good oral
health as a preventive measure for throat infections.

____

____

____

____

____

____

____

____

____

____

❖ How do you prioritize oral hygiene in preventing
tonsillitis? Discuss the importance of maintaining good oral
health as a preventive measure for throat infections.

____

____

____

____

____

____

____

____

____

____

Spinal Meningitis

❖ How would you explain spinal meningitis to someone unfamiliar with the condition? Share any experiences or knowledge you have regarding the causes and symptoms of this inflammation.

____

____

____

____

____

____

____

____

____

❖ Explore the role of vaccination in preventing spinal meningitis. What are your thoughts on vaccination as a preventive measure, and how do you approach discussions about vaccines for serious infections?

____

____

____

____

____

____

____

____

❖ Delve into the herbal remedies mentioned for supporting
  the immune system against spinal meningitis, such as
  garlic. Have you tried any of these herbs, and how do you
  integrate them into your routine? Share your experiences
  with herbal support for immune health.

____

____

____

____

____

____

____

____

____

Malaria

❖ How familiar are you with malaria? Share any prior
  knowledge or experiences you have regarding this
  mosquito-borne disease.

____

____

____

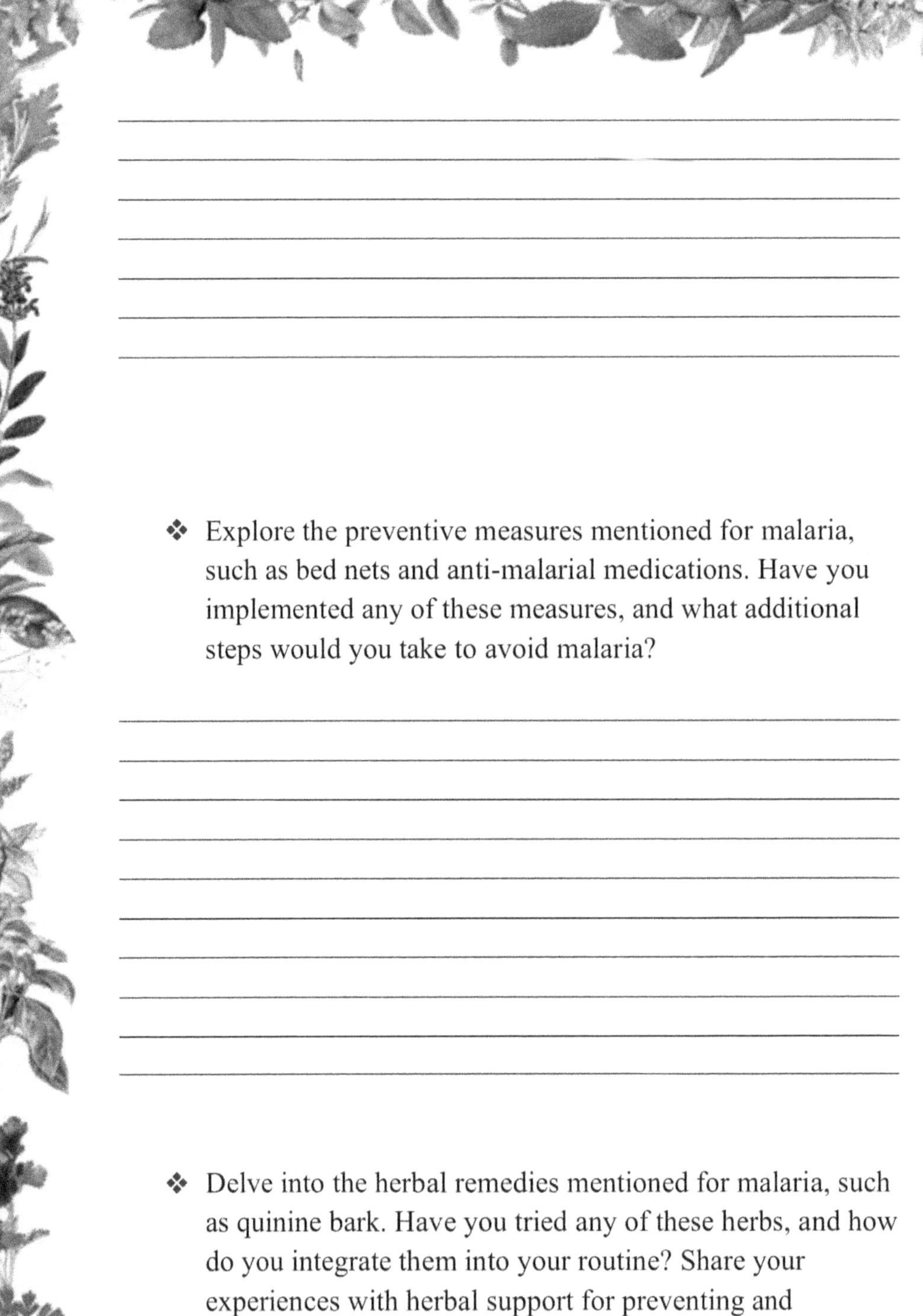

❖ Explore the preventive measures mentioned for malaria, such as bed nets and anti-malarial medications. Have you implemented any of these measures, and what additional steps would you take to avoid malaria?

❖ Delve into the herbal remedies mentioned for malaria, such as quinine bark. Have you tried any of these herbs, and how do you integrate them into your routine? Share your experiences with herbal support for preventing and managing malaria.

Tuberculosis

❖ How familiar are you with tuberculosis? Share any prior knowledge or experiences you have regarding this bacterial infection.

____

❖ Early diagnosis is crucial in managing tuberculosis. What steps would you take or suggest if someone shows symptoms of this condition? Discuss the importance of prompt medical attention.

____
____
____
____
____
____
____
____
____

❖ Adherence to prescribed medications is vital in managing tuberculosis. How do you approach discussions about medication adherence with others? Share your understanding of the challenges and importance of compliance with tuberculosis treatment.

____
____
____
____
____
____
____
____
____

Syphilis

❖ How familiar are you with syphilis? Share any prior knowledge or experiences you have regarding this sexually transmitted infection.

____
____
____
____
____
____

❖ Discuss the importance of safe sexual practices in preventing syphilis. How do you approach conversations about sexual health and the use of protection with others? Share your perspectives on sexual education.

____
____
____
____
____
____

❖ Regular screening is recommended for sexually active individuals to detect syphilis early. How do you approach discussions about the importance of regular STI screenings? Discuss the role of awareness and testing in preventing the spread of syphilis.

____

____

____

____

____

____

❖ When it comes to sexually transmitted infections like syphilis, have you explored or heard about herbal remedies? Share any insights, personal experiences, or anecdotes related to using herbs for sexual health and well-being.

____

____

____

____

____

____

Gonorrhea

❖ In addressing sexually transmitted infections like gonorrhea, have you explored or considered herbal remedies? Share personal stories, insights, or experiences related to using herbs for sexual health and overall well-being.

____

____

____

____

____

____

❖ How comfortable are you discussing the role of herbs like wormwood, black walnut hulls, and cloves in promoting safe practices and preventing gonorrhea? Share your thoughts on incorporating herbal preventatives into personal and community health practices.

____

____

____

____

____

❖ If given the chance, would you actively participate in community discussions about herbal solutions for sexual health, including managing gonorrhea? Discuss your views on the importance of open conversations and herbal education in such contexts.

____
____
____
____
____
____

Fever

❖ When it comes to managing fever, have you explored or considered herbal remedies? Share personal stories, insights, or experiences related to using herbs for fever relief and overall well-being.

____
____
____
____
____
____
____

❖ How comfortable are you incorporating herbs like agrimony, vervain, boneset, and culver's root into herbal teas for managing fever? Share your thoughts on the comfort and effectiveness of herbal teas during febrile conditions.

____

____

____

____

____

____

____

____

❖ In your personal circles, how do you share herbal wisdom for managing fever at home? Share personal anecdotes or advice on using herbal remedies for comfort and relief during periods of elevated body temperature

____

____

____

____

____

____

____

PART X: DERMATOLOGICAL CONDITIONS

This chapter is dedicated to understanding and incorporating herbal remedies for various skin conditions. In this exploration, we delve into the efficacy of herbs in addressing concerns like acne, dandruff, eczema, scabies, burns, bed sores, and more. Feel free to engage and share your personal stories. Let's embark on a journey of herbal wellness and discover the power of nature's solutions for your skin.

Every skin Condition

❖ Have you ever ventured into using herbal remedies for common skin conditions? Share your experiences or any herbal solutions you've explored to address issues like irritation, redness, or dryness on your skin.

____

____

____

____

____

____

____

____

____

❖ How comfortable are you incorporating herbs like aloe vera, calendula, or chamomile into your daily skincare routine? Share personal anecdotes or tips on seamlessly integrating herbal remedies into your skincare practices.

❖ If you were to exchange herbal wisdom with friends or family for overall skin health, what specific herbs or natural ingredients would you recommend? Discuss your favorite herbal remedies for maintaining healthy and radiant skin.

____

____

____

____

____

____

____

____

____

____

____

____

____

Skin Ulcer

❖ When faced with skin ulcers or wounds, have you explored or heard about herbal remedies? Share any personal healing journeys or insights related to using herbs for promoting skin recovery and minimizing scarring.

____

____

____

____

____

____

____

____

____

❖ How comfortable are you discussing the role of herbs like comfrey, echinacea, or calendula in providing comfort and aiding the healing process for skin ulcers? Share your thoughts on incorporating these herbs into personal and community first aid practices.

____

____

____

____

____

____

____

____

❖ If you were to share a personal story about using herbal remedies for skin ulcer recovery, what would it be? Share anecdotes or advice based on your experiences with herbal solutions during the healing process.

____

____

____

____

____

____

____

____

____

____

Burns and Carbuncle

❖ In times of burns or carbuncles, have you explored herbal remedies for immediate relief and recovery? Share personal stories, insights, or experiences related to using herbs like aloe vera, lavender, or chamomile for burn management.

____

____

____

____

____

____

____

❖ How comfortable are you discussing the role of herbs like plantain, calendula, or St. John's wort in providing comfort and aiding the healing process for burns and carbuncles? Share your thoughts on incorporating these herbs into personal and community first aid practices.

❖ If given the chance to share a healing moment involving herbal remedies for burns or carbuncles, what would your story be? Share personal anecdotes or advice based on your experiences with herbal solutions during the recovery process.

Bed Sores

❖ Have you ever explored herbal remedies for preventing or managing bed sores? Share any personal stories, insights, or experiences related to using herbs like arnica, calendula, or chamomile to care for sensitive skin areas.

❖ How comfortable are you incorporating herbs like lavender, comfrey, or aloe vera into daily care routines to prevent bed sores? Share personal anecdotes or tips on seamlessly integrating herbal remedies into personal care practices.

❖ If you were to impart herbal wisdom for those with sensitive skin prone to bed sores, what specific herbs or natural practices would you recommend? Discuss your favorite herbal remedies for maintaining skin health in vulnerable areas.

Eczema

❖ When dealing with eczema, have you explored or considered herbal remedies? Share personal stories, insights, or experiences related to using herbs like calendula, chamomile, or chickweed for eczema management.

____

____

____

____

____

____

____

____

❖ How comfortable are you discussing the role of herbs like licorice root, borage, or lavender in soothing irritated skin and managing eczema? Share your thoughts on incorporating herbal remedies into personal skincare practices.

____

____

____

____

____

____

❖ If given the chance, would you actively participate in community discussions about herbal solutions for eczema? Discuss your views on the importance of open conversations and herbal education in promoting holistic skincare practices.

Scabies

❖ Have you ever ventured into using herbal remedies for managing scabies? Share your experiences or any herbal solutions you've explored to address the symptoms and discomfort associated with scabies.

❖ How comfortable are you discussing the role of herbs like neem, tea tree oil, or calendula in soothing irritated skin and managing scabies? Share your thoughts on incorporating these herbs into personal and community care practices.

❖ If you were to share a personal solution involving herbal remedies for scabies, what would it be? Share anecdotes or advice based on your experiences with herbal solutions during the management of scabies.

PART XI: REPRODUCTIVE AND GYNELOGICAL DISORDERS

Welcome to a chapter dedicated to exploring the realm of herbal remedies in the context of reproductive and gynecological health. In this journey, we unravel the nuanced aspects of endometriosis, erectile dysfunction, and polycystic ovary syndrome (PCOS). Engage in personal reflections, shared insights, and envision a future where herbal remedies seamlessly complement conventional approaches. Let's embark on a holistic exploration of well-being, celebrating the wisdom of nature in the realm of reproductive health.

Endometriosis

* ❖ Have you or someone you know experienced endometriosis, and what impact did it have on daily life?

____

____

____

____

____

____

____

____

____

❖ Share your thoughts on how herbal remedies might complement traditional treatments for managing endometriosis symptoms.

____

____

____

____

____

____

____

____

____

❖ How might incorporating herbal teas or tinctures into your routine positively influence your overall well-being while dealing with endometriosis?

____

____

____

____

____

____

____

____

____

Erectie Dysfunction

❖ In what ways has erectile dysfunction affected relationships or personal confidence, either directly or indirectly in your life?

____

____

____

____

____

____

____

____

____

____

❖ Discuss any preconceptions or experiences you have with herbal remedies for addressing erectile dysfunction.

____

____

____

____

____

____

____

____

____

❖ How do you envision incorporating herbal solutions into your daily life to support overall reproductive health?

____

____

____

____

____

____

____

____

Polycystic Ovary Syndrome

❖ If you or someone close has faced PCOS, share the challenges encountered and the impact on mental and emotional well-being.

____

____

____

____

____

____

____

____

❖ Explore your understanding of how herbal remedies could potentially provide relief or support for PCOS symptoms

____

____

____

____

____

____

____

____

❖ How committed are you to making lifestyle changes, including the integration of herbal remedies, to manage or alleviate PCOS-related concerns?

____

____

____

____

____

____

____

____

____

PART XII: OTHER CONDITIONS

This chapter narrows its attention to a variety of other conditions from cataracts to infectious diseases like bird flu, and common illnesses like vomiting and nausea. It also extends to childhood illnesses like measles, mumps and whooping cough, with serious conditions like typhoid, fever, cholera and tetanus. Keep engaging!

Cataracts

❖ Have you or someone you know faced challenges related to cataracts? Share any personal experiences or insights into how this condition impacts daily life.

____

____

____

____

____

____

____

____

❖ Reflect on your perceptions of herbal remedies in supporting eye health.

____

____

____

____

____

____

____

____

____

Bird Flu

❖ Discuss your level of awareness about bird flu and its
potential impact on health. How might herbal remedies
play a role in prevention or management from your
perspective?

____

____

____

____

____

____

____

____

____

____

❖ Share any knowledge or experiences you have with the
recommended herbs known for immune system support and
their potential effectiveness against viral infections.

Nausea and Vomitting

❖ How do you personally deal with episodes of nausea and vomiting? Consider the potential benefits of herbal remedies in alleviating these symptoms.

❖ Share any herbal solutions or remedies you've heard about or tried for managing nausea. What role do you envision them playing in your well-being?

Small Pox

❖ Have you ever had small pox before? If yes, share your experiences.

❖ Share any herbal solutions or remedies you've heard about or tried for managing nausea. What role do you envision them playing in your well-being?

____
____
____
____

Measles, Mumps and Whooping Cough

❖ Share any personal experiences or encounters with measles, mumps, or whooping cough.

____
____
____
____
____
____
____
____
____

❖ How do these childhood illnesses shape your perception of herbal remedies in maintaining immune health?

____
____
____
____

Typhoid, Cholera and Tetanus

❖ Share any personal experiences or encounters with measles, mumps, or whooping cough. How do these childhood illnesses shape your perception of herbal remedies in maintaining immune health?

❖ Discuss your understanding of the global impact of diseases like typhoid fever, cholera, and tetanus. How might herbal

remedies contribute to preventive measures or supportive
care?

____

____

____

____

____

____

____

____

____

____

____

____

____

PART XIII: COMPREHENSIVE GUIDE TO PAIN MANAGEMENT

This chapter delves into the realm of comprehensive pain management through herbal remedies. From toe and finger pain to arthritis and inflammation, share your personal insights and experiences. Let's collectively explore the efficacy of herbal remedies in crafting a holistic approach to pain relief.

Toe and Finger Pain

❖ Share any personal experiences or anecdotes related to toe or finger pain.

____
____
____
____
____
____
____
____

❖ How did it impact your daily life, and have you explored herbal remedies for relief?

____
____
____
____
____
____
____
____

❖ If you've considered herbal remedies, which specific herbs or natural solutions have you found effective in managing toe or finger pain?

Lumbago

❖ Discuss the impact of lower back pain on your daily activities.

❖ Have you explored herbal remedies to alleviate lumbago, and if so, share your experiences and insights?

❖ Explore herbal combinations that you believe may be effective in managing lower back pain. How do these align with your overall approach to pain management?

Osteoarthritis and Rheumatoid arthritis

❖ Share your strategies for managing pain associated with arthritis. Have herbal remedies played a role in your approach, and if yes, which ones have you found beneficial?

____

____

____

____

____

____

____

____

____

❖ Discuss your vision for achieving long-term relief from arthritis pain. How do herbal remedies fit into your holistic approach to managing arthritis?

____

____

____

____

____

____

____

____

Prostate Gland Inflammation

❖ Reflect on the personal impact of prostate gland inflammation on your well-being. Have you considered herbal remedies, and if so, how have they contributed to your pain management plan?

____

____

____

____

____

____

____

____

____

____

❖ Explore specific herbs known for promoting prostate health. How do these herbs align with your overall strategy for managing inflammation and discomfort?

____

____

____

____

____

____

____

____

____

Mouth Sores

❖ Have you ever had mouth sores? Discuss the challenges
posed by mouth sores in your daily life.

❖ Have you explored herbal remedies for relief, and if yes,
share your experiences and any go-to remedies you've
discovered?

❖ Explore herbal solutions for oral health. How do these remedies contribute to your comprehensive approach to managing mouth sores?

____

____

____

____

____

____

____

____

____

Eye Pain

❖ Share how eye pain or ache has impacted your vision and daily activities. Have you considered herbal remedies to alleviate eye discomfort, and if so, which ones have you found effective?

❖ Discuss your herbal eye care routine. How do you integrate
herbs into your daily practices for maintaining eye health?

Prostate Enlargement

❖ Reflect on the challenges of dealing with prostate
enlargement. How have herbal remedies factored into your
pain management and overall well-being?

❖ Explore herbs known for supporting prostate health. How do these herbs contribute to your proactive approach in managing enlargement-related discomfort?

Ear Ache

❖ Discuss how earaches have impacted your daily life and activities. Have you sought relief through herbal remedies, and if so, share your experiences and any herbal solutions you find effective?

____

____

____

____

____

____

____

____

____

____

____

____

____

❖ Explore herbal practices for ear health. How do these remedies fit into your holistic approach to managing earaches?

____

____

____

____

____

____

____

____

____

PART XIV: OVERCOMING SPECIFIC HEALTH CHALLENGES (NON-PAINFUL DISEASES)

Diabetes

❖ Share your understanding of diabetes. How has this health condition impacted your life or the lives of those around you?

____

____

____

____

____

____

____

____

____

____

____

____

____

____

____

____

____

____

____

❖ Explore your knowledge of herbal remedies for diabetes.
How do you envision incorporating herbs into your
diabetes management?

❖ Name specific herbs you believe could be beneficial for diabetes. How do you envision including them in your meals or routines?

____

____

____

____

____

____

____

❖ Reflect on your journey of learning about diabetes and herbal remedies. What educational resources have been helpful, and how have they empowered you?

____

____

____

____

____

____

____

Worms9 Infestation

❖ Share any personal encounters with worms' infestation.
   How did it impact your health and daily life?

____

____

____

____

____

____

____

❖ Discuss any symptoms you've experienced during worms'
   infestation. How did these symptoms prompt you to
   explore herbal remedies?

____

____

____

____

____

____

____

____

❖ Name herbs you believe could offer relief from worms'
   infestation. How might these herbs address specific
   symptoms?

____

____

____

____

Dysentery

❖ Share any personal experiences with dysentery. How did it affect your daily life and overall well-being?

❖ Discuss any symptoms you've experienced during dysentery. How did these symptoms prompt you to explore herbal remedies?

❖ Name herbs you believe could offer relief from dysentery.
How might these herbs address specific symptoms?

____

____

____

____

____

____

____

❖ Discuss actions you take or plan to take to prevent
dysentery. How do herbal remedies fit into your preventive
measures?

____

____

____

____

____

____

____

Insomnia

❖ Share insights into your sleep patterns and any experiences
with insomnia. How does insomnia impact your daily life
and overall well-being?

____

____

____

❖ Discuss specific challenges you face when dealing with insomnia. How do these challenges influence your exploration of herbal remedies?

❖ Name herbs you believe could offer support in managing insomnia. How might these herbs address specific sleep challenges?

❖ Share any herbal practices related to managing sleep
challenges within your family or community. How arc
these remedies shared and passed down?

____

____

____

____

____

____

____

Burns and Injuries

❖ Share any personal encounters with burns or injuries. How
did they impact your health and daily life?

____

____

____

____

____

____

____

❖ Share insights into your first aid practices for burns and
injuries. How might herbs be integrated into your first aid
kit for immediate relief?

____

____

____

❖ Discuss how you envision incorporating herbs into your routine for long-term recovery from burns and injuries.

Hiccups

❖ Share any personal experiences with hiccups. How do frequent hiccups impact your daily life and overall well-being?

❖ Discuss specific triggers for your hiccups. How do these triggers influence your exploration of herbal remedies?

❖ Discuss actions you take or plan to take to prevent hiccups. How do herbal remedies fit into your preventive measures?

Constipation

❖ Share your experiences in dealing with constipation. How has it impacted your daily life and overall well-being?

❖ Discuss specific triggers for your constipation. How do these triggers influence your exploration of herbal remedies?

❖ Name herbs you believe could offer support for bowel health. How might these herbs address specific triggers of constipation?

Night sweats, Nervousness and Bed Wetting

❖ Have you or someone you know dealt with any of these
   health issues?

❖ Reflect on personal experiences with symptoms related to
   these health issues.

❖ Explore any herbal remedies that are associated with these
   conditions.

PART XV: SPECIALIZED HEALING TECHNIQUES

Fasting and its healing effects

❖ Have you ever considered or practiced fasting for health benefits? If so, what was your experience?

____

____

____

____

____

____

____

❖ How do you perceive the synergy between fasting and herbal medicine in promoting overall health and well-being?

____

____

____

____

____

____

____

❖ Reflect on the statement, Sometimes, the most effective medicine is the kind that has existed in nature all along.= How does this resonate with your views on health?

____
____
____
____
____
____
____
____

Hydrotheray and its uses

- ❖ Have you ever experienced hydrotherapy treatments? If so, how did it make you feel, and did you notice any positive effects on your well-being?

____
____
____
____
____
____
____

- ❖ In your opinion, how does the infusion of herbal properties into hydrotherapy enhance the overall therapeutic experience?

____
____
____
____

____

____

____

____

❖ Reflect on the statement, "Herbs can alleviate symptoms of anxiety and depression, promote relaxation, and improve sleep quality, addressing the mind-body connection in healing." How do you perceive this mind-body connection in your well-being?

____

____

____

____

____

____

____

____

❖ How open are you to exploring natural healing methods like hydrotherapy and herbal medicine alongside conventional approaches to holistic health?

____

____

____

The Benefits of Reflexology and Acupressure

- ❖ Have you ever tried reflexology or acupressure? If yes, how did it impact your well-being? If not, would you consider trying these techniques in the future?

- ❖ Reflect on the statement, "Modern medicine often targets symptoms, providing quick fixes rather than addressing the root cause of ailments. Reflexology and acupressure seek to harmonize the body's natural balance." What are your thoughts on this difference in approach?

❖ In what ways do you believe herbs can influence the effectiveness of reflexology and acupressure in supporting and enhancing the body's natural healing processes?

Chiropathic and Osteopathic Approaches to Health

❖ Have you ever experience or learned about chiropathic or osteopathic approaches to health? If yes, what was your impression? If not, how open are you to exploring these practices

❖ Consider anti-inflammatory herbs like turmeric or ginger. How do you envision those herbs complementing chiropathic treatments to enhance the body's recovery?

❖ In what ways does the integration of herbs in chiropathic and osteopathic practices contribute to a more comprehensive understanding of health and healing?

PART XVI: LIFESTYLE FOR LONGEVITY AND WELLNESS

The Importance of a Healthy Diet

❖ What does a healthy diet mean to you?

____

____

____

____

____

____

____

❖ How has your awareness or understanding of herbs evolved after learning about their holistic benefits in supporting the body's natural healing processes?

____

____

____

____

____

____

____

____

❖ How do you plan to incorporate herbs into your daily diet as a way to improve your health?

____

____

❖ What challenges do you often face in finding the right herbs that work for you?

The Role of Mental and Emotional Well-being

❖ In your understanding, state how herbs work to improve our mental and emotional well-being?

❖ What challenges do you often face while finding the right herbs that work for you?

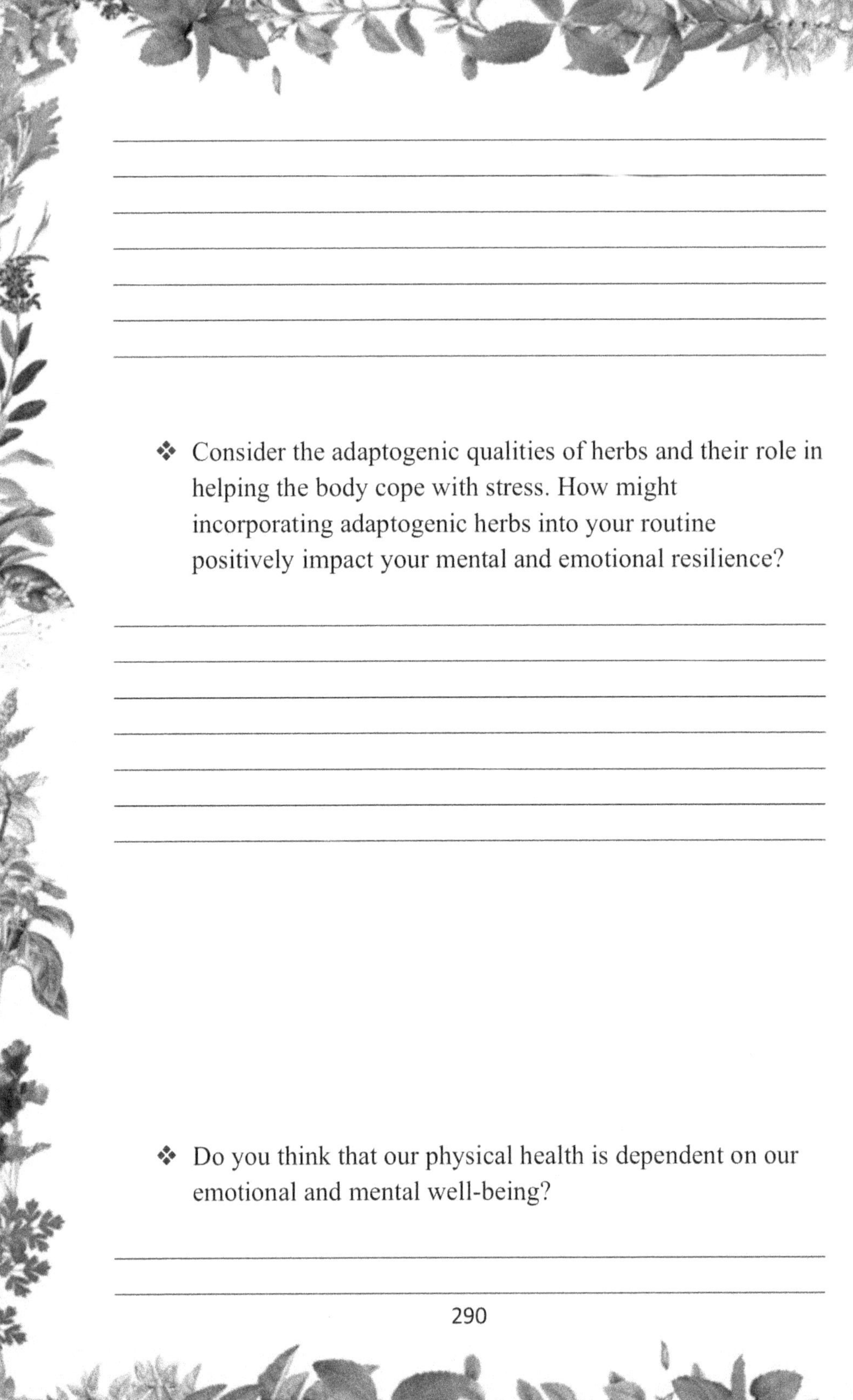

❖ Consider the adaptogenic qualities of herbs and their role in helping the body cope with stress. How might incorporating adaptogenic herbs into your routine positively impact your mental and emotional resilience?

❖ Do you think that our physical health is dependent on our emotional and mental well-being?

❖ Share your thoughts on the influence of the pharmaceutical industry on the perception of herbal remedies. How can awareness be raised to ensure a more unbiased view of the benefits herbs offer in mental and emotional well-being?

❖ How much impact do you think that the right use of herbs will have in our longevity and wellness as opposed to the use of synthetic drugs?

Cultivating Daily Routines for Optimal Health

❖ Reflect on your current sleep habits. How might prioritizing both the quality and quantity of sleep positively impact your mental and physical well-being?

❖ Consider the role of herbs like turmeric, ginger, and garlic in daily nutrition. How can you seamlessly integrate these herbs into your meals to enhance their health benefits?

❖ Explore your current physical activity routine. What enjoyable and approachable activities could you incorporate into your daily life to improve cardiovascular health, flexibility, and stress levels?

❖ Evaluate your engagement in mental health practices like meditation or mindfulness. How might incorporating such practices contribute to stress reduction and overall mental well-being?

____

____

____

____

____

____

____

____

____

____

____

____

____

❖ Reflect on the strength of your social connections. In what ways can you nurture and expand your social ties to enhance emotional support, reduce stress, and cultivate a sense of belonging?

____

____

____

____

____

____

____

❖ Consider the idea of building healthy habits that resonate with your individual needs and lifestyle. What small, consistent changes can you make to align your daily routine with your overall well-being goals?

Cultivate a Healthy Living Environment

❖ Reflect on your living space. How can you enhance air quality, considering ventilation, air purifiers, and indoor plants? How might this contribute to better respiratory health?

❖ Consider your water consumption habits. In what ways can you ensure clean, filtered water for drinking and cooking? How might investing in a water filtration system positively impact your long-term health?

❖ Explore your dietary preferences. How can you shift towards a whole-food, plant-based diet enriched with herbs like turmeric, ginger, and garlic to promote immunity and overall health?

❖ Evaluate your physical activity routine. How can you incorporate regular exercise, whether through walking, yoga, or other activities, to improve cardiovascular health and reduce stress?

❖ Examine your current mental health practices. In what ways can you integrate meditation, mindfulness, or nature engagement to reduce stress and enhance overall mental well-being?

❖ Assess your sleep environment. How can you create a more sleep-conducive space, considering factors like darkness, quietness, and coolness? What changes can you make to improve sleep quality?

❖ Reflect on your social connections. How can you actively engage in community activities, nurture relationships, and seek positive social interactions to foster a supportive environment for health and longevity?

❖ Consider the multifaceted nature of creating a healthy living environment. How can you integrate physical, dietary, mental, and social aspects into your daily life to promote vitality, wellness, and longevity?

CONCLUSION

Embracing self-healing in daily life isn't just a journey; it's a transformative tapestry woven into our existence for holistic health. Our bodies are strongly, inherently equipped for self-healing to find support in the wisdom of herbs. This is a strong truth which is often overlooked yet central to our well-being.

Herbs are versatile and accessible. They offer practicality in everyday health, from chamomile's calm to echinacea's immunity. Yet, this holistic journey is perpetual, touching mental, emotional, and spiritual facets. It's a personal expedition, requiring patience, experimentation, and deep listening to our body's signals.

In essence, concluding this exploration isn't an end but an ongoing invitation. Trust your body's wisdom, delve into the world of herbs, and nurture vibrant health and harmony within yourself and with the natural world. The journey is not just about treating illnesses but about fostering a state of vibrant well-being.

Lastly, you are encouraged to go over the reflections and exercises with regards to the health issue you want to explore. Be open and engage it. I wish you all the best on your purposeful path to wellness.

www.ingramcontent.com/pod-product-compliance
Lightning Source LLC
Chambersburg PA
CBHW052355030726

47599CB00014B/1066